Atlas of
Trans-Oesophageal Echocardiography

An Anaesthesiologist's Perspective

Atlas of
Trans-Oesophageal Echocardiography
An Anaesthesiologist's Perspective

Deepak K. Tempe, MD

Professor & Head
Department of Anaesthesiology & Intensive Care,
G.B. Pant Hospital (University of Delhi)
New Delhi - 110002

Partho P. Sengupta, MD, DM

Post-doctoral Research Fellow,
Division of Cardiovascular Disease and Internal Medicine
Mayo Clinic, Rochester,
MN, U.S.A.

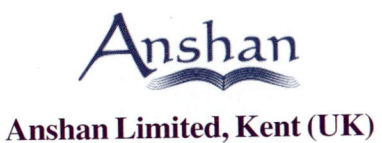

Anshan Limited, Kent (UK)

Anshan Limited
6 Newlands Road
Tunbridge Wells
Kent TN4 9AT
UK

Tel/Fax: +44 (0) 1892 557767
e-mail:info@anshan.co.uk
Web site: www.anshan.co.uk

This edition of Deepak K Tempe and Partho P Sengupta : *Atlas of Trans-oesophageal echocardiography - An Anaesthesiologist's Perspective*, is published by arrangement with B.I. Publications Pvt Ltd, 54, Janpath, New Delhi – 110001 (India).

British Library Cataloguing in Publication Data
A catalogue record for this book is available from the British Library

Not for sale in India, Pakistan, Nepal, Sri Lanka and Bangladesh

ISBN 1-904798-23-3

The UK Edition is published by Anshan Limited and printed at Saurabh Printers Pvt. Ltd., NOIDA, India

To Anuradha, my daughter, who has willfully allowed the utilisation of my time that belonged to her.

Deepak K. Tempe

I dedicate this atlas to the memory of my father, the Late. Dr. Pradeep Kumar Sengupta.

Partho P. Sengupta

Foreword

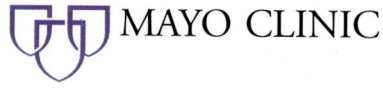 MAYO CLINIC

200 First Street SW
Rochester, MN 55905
507-284-2511

Bijoy K. Khandheria, M.D.
Cardiovascular Diseases
& Internal Medicine

This TOE atlas written by Dr. Deepak K. Tempe and Dr. Partho P. Sengupta represents academic excellence in the field of trans-oesphageal echocardiography. This is not a textbook but an atlas that should and must be used by those practicing TOE. The fundamentals are easy to read and depicted in a format that is "easy" reading. The images should lend a helping hand to the practitioners. Echocardiographers and anaesthesiologists alike should find this atlas useful in their clinical practice.

I commend the authors for having done an excellent job of putting together this pictorial depiction. The herculean task will be rewarded by the readers as they improve the practice of echocardiography using knowledge gained from this atlas.

It is my privilege to have been asked to write a foreword for this book.

Good Luck to the readers. Congratulations to the writers.

Bijoy K Khandheria, MD. FACC
Professor of Medicine
Mayo Medical School
Consultant Cardiovascular Disease and Internal Medicine
Mayo Clinic

Preface

The advances in the ultrasound technology and its application for examining the heart and great vessels have revolutionized the field of diagnostic cardiology. The introduction of trans-oesophageal echocardiography (TOE) in clinical practice further widened the scope of echocardiography and also entered the cardiac operating theatre. The TOE allowed continuous observation of the heart during operations without interfering with the surgical field. This offered the anaesthesiologist with the possibility of looking at the on-line dynamic images of heart dimensions and function. The opportunity was grabbed with open hands by the anaesthesiologist who till recently, at best, was satisfied with monitoring the patient's pressures and flows. TOE soon became an indispensable part of cardiac surgery, with cardiac surgeons increasingly relying on it, to form the basis of important intraoperative decisions.

The cardiologists were not always available to perform TOE in the operating theatre, which resulted in the anaesthesiologist taking over the responsibility. We firmly believe (like most others) that TOE has a significant impact on the outcome of patient. Today, many anaesthesiologists have learned the specialised technique and the cardiac surgeon is appreciative of this fact and often looks forward to knowing important findings that assist him in taking crucial surgical decisions. This has largely influenced the number of patients having to undergo another cardiac surgery because of residual defects or other significant abnormalities remaining undetected during the first operation. The anaesthesiologist of course, utilises the haemodynamic data derived from the TOE to choose the best pharmacological intervention for his patient. This new role of the cardiac anaesthesiologist was achieved in a close and fruitful cooperation with the cardiologists.

It is often questioned whether the anaesthesiologist can manage a complicated or critical anaesthesia and at the same time perform TOE. In this respect, it should be accepted that at times, it may be necessary to have a second anaesthesiologist who takes charge of the anaesthetic management while the TOE is being performed. In addition, there will always be situations when assistance from a cardiologist will be needed. This approach is welcome and is a common practice in our institution.

In the western world, the TOE entered the cardiac operating theatres in the late 80s, and in India in late 90s. There is growing need to impart TOE as a part of the training process of all the cardiac anaesthesiologists so that the same can be utilised for the patient care. In this respect, it was felt that understanding of the images is of immense importance and that an atlas demonstrating the normal as well as the commonly encountered abnormal images would be helpful. The atlas has been prepared with this objective in mind, with the hope that it will facilitate the understanding of this relatively new subject. I sincerely hope that the reader will find it useful.

I must acknowledge the department of Anaesthesiology and Intensive care, G.B. Pant Hospital, New Delhi, where I have acquired most of my experience in cardiac anaesthesia. I should also thank all my colleagues (faculty as well as residents) in the department, who have worked together like a family and always provided an atmosphere suitable for carrying out this work. Special thanks are due to Dr. Partho Sengupta, who has worked tirelessly with me in preparation of this atlas. This involved choosing the best images, (from the large collection that I had acquired over 2 years) and writing appropriate legends. I gratefully acknowledge the department of Cardiothoracic Surgery and its staff members for their cooperation in carrying out this work. Although, there are many who have been my well wishers and encouraged me at every step, a few names deserve a special mention. They are Dr. Veena Malhotra, Dr. A.K. Singh, Dr. Yatin Mehta, Dr. Rajiv Juneja and Dr. Vijay Trehan.

Lastly, I must thank Anjali (my wife) and Anuradha (my daughter) for their consistent support and patience during preparation of this book.

I acknowledge the efforts of Mr. YR Chadha and Mr. Aman Sachdeva of the BI Publications and M/s Saurabh Printers Pvt. Ltd. for publishing the book in a very short time.

Deepak K. Tempe

Preface

Anaesthesia during cardiothoracic surgery has become increasingly complex since several diverse set of cardiac problems currently undergo surgical correction. Although a variety of modalities are available for assessing cardiac function and haemodynamics, trans-oesophageal echocardiography (TOE) has been increasingly used by cardiologists and cardiac-anaesthetists for making critical therapeutic decisions in the perioperative period. However performance and interpretation of TOE has a significant learning curve and needs expertise. The role of an atlas therefore assumes significance since a pictorial overview of transesophageal techniques can quickly familiarize a beginner to commonly encountered problems in day to day practice while performing TOE in the operating room.

"...to suppress the pictures is to suppress a powerful source of suggestion... Pictorial representation is essential for discovery and rapid understanding.....J.L. Synge in The Hypercircle in Mathematical Physics (1957)"

The idea to compile an atlas conceptualized during my stay as a Senior Research Associate in the Department of Cardiology, G.B. Pant Hospital and stands as a testimonial to the support and co-operation I enjoyed at an important stage of my career. I feel honoured in having an invitation from Prof. Tempe to be a co-author of this atlas. I have always admired his zeal, enthusiasm and meticulous efforts in undertaking any scientific endeavor, and I feel privileged in having this opportunity to work with him. I need to specially thank Prof. JC Mohan, whose support and motivation proved vital from time to time, and whom I consider responsible for developing in me a quest for academic pursuits. It was also an enormous privilege to have closely interacted with faculty members and fellows at G.B. Pant Hospital who were always more than willing to help me and whose experiences contributed enormously to my understanding of the subject of cardiology. I thank my family and my friends for their love, affection and their whole-hearted support. At this juncture it would also be befitting for me to pay my humble regards to my spiritual master for his blessings and guidance that helped awaken in me the 'true values' of life.

'I expect to pass through life but once. If therefore, there be any kindness I can show, or any good thing I can do to any fellow being, let me do it now, and not defer or neglect it, as I shall not pass this way again.' - William Penn

Partho P. Sengupta

Contents

Foreword by Bijoy K. Khandheria .... *vii*

Preface by Dr. Deepak K. Tempe .... *ix*

Preface by Dr. Partho P. Sengupta .... *xi*

1. Principles of echocardiography 1
2. Cardiac assessment 7
3. Evaluation of the left ventricular function 39
4. Evaluation of the mitral valve 53
5. Evaluation of the aortic valve 75
6. Evaluation of the right side of the heart 89
7. Evaluation of the prosthetic valve function 103
8. Assessment of cardiac vegetations 117
9. Evaluation of congenital heart disease 123
10. Evaluation of the intra-cardiac masses and prosthetic materials 147
11. Evaluation of the aorta 169
12. Further Reading 176

List of Abbreviations

AA	Ascending aorta
ALPM	Anterolateral papillary muscle
AML	Anterior mitral leaflet
AO	Aorta
ASD	Atrial septal defect
AV	Aortic valve
CS	Coronary sinus
IAS	Interatrial septum
IVC	Inferior vena cava
IVS	Interventricular septum
LA	Left atrium
LAA	Left atrial appendage
LAD	Left anterior descending artery
LCX	Left circumflex artery
LCC	Left coronary cusp
LPV	Left upper pulmonary vein
LSVC	Left superior vena cava
LV	Left ventricle
LVOT	Left ventricular outflow tract
MR	Mitral regurgitation
MV	Mitral valve
NCC	Non coronary cusp
PA	Pulmonary artery
PML	Posterior mitral leaflet
PMPM	Posteromedial papillary muscle
RA	Right atrium
RAA	Right atrial appendage
RCA	Right coronary artery
RCC	Right coronary cusp
RSOV	Ruptured sinus of Valsalva
RUPV	Right upper pulmonary vein
RV	Right ventricle
RVOT	Right ventricular outflow tract
SEC	Spontaneous echo contrast
SVC	Superior vena cava
TOE	Trans-oesophageal echocardiography
TV	Tricuspid valve
VSD	Ventricular septal defect

Chapter 1

PRINCIPLES OF ECHOCARDIOGRAPHY

Echocardiography in the operating room was introduced in the 1970s and the use of trans-oesophageal echocardiography (TOE) during surgery was first described in 1980. Its application grew subsequently with technical developments in high-frequency transducers and colour Doppler imaging. The physical principles and instrumentation of TOE involve concepts similar to those of surface echocardiography and are briefly outlined in this chapter.

Physical properties of ultrasound

The frequency of ultrasonic waves is above the audible range of the human ear and exceeds 20,000 cycles/sec. They can be directed in a beam and obey laws of reflection and refraction (Figure 1.1). Waves reflected at the interphase between two materials with different densities are used for forming an image. Ultrasonic waves propagate freely in liquids, but very poorly through air. They are almost completely reflected by dense substances like metal, calcium or bone. Penetration also depends on the frequency of incidental wave; higher the frequency poorer the penetration although the near-resolution is superior. A reduction in resolution occurs with increasing depth and is called as attenuation. In human body, the total depth that can be travelled by ultrasound is about one-fourth of the wavelength of ultrasound. In a trans-oesophageal examination, heart is close to the transducer with little intervening tissues, the frequency used (3.5-5 MHz) therefore, is higher than that required for trans-thoracic examination in adults (2-3.5 MHz).

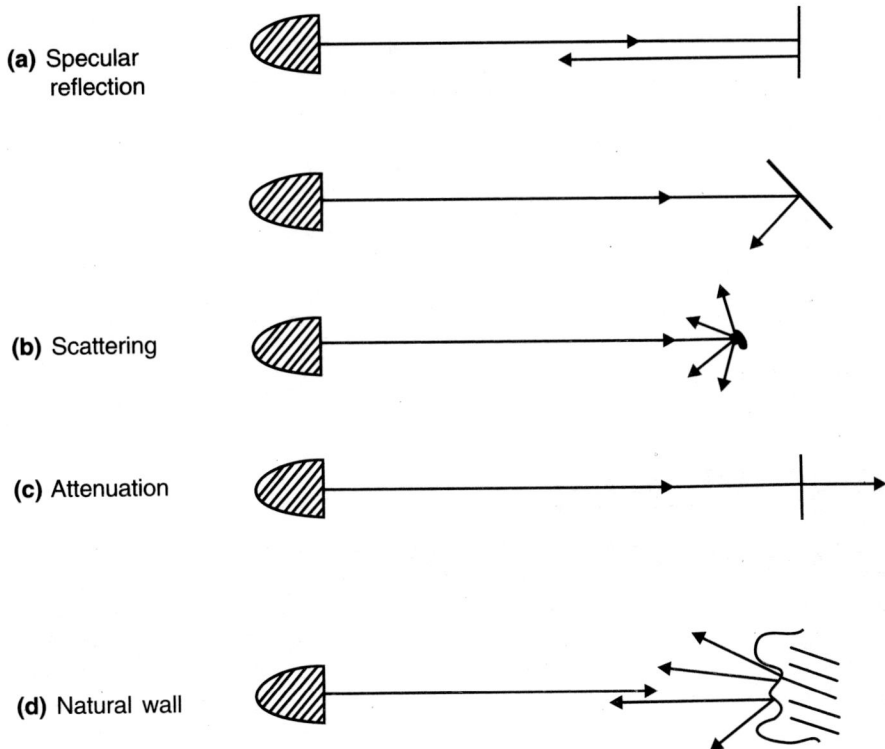

(a) Specular reflection

(b) Scattering

(c) Attenuation

(d) Natural wall

Figure 1.1. Patterns of interference between an ultrasound wave and a target. Natural structures are inhomogenous and behave as a mixture of specular (a), scattering (b) and attenuation (c).

Production of ultrasound and transducers

In clinical practice ultrasonic waves are produced from piezo-electric crystals. These crystals change their shape in electric fields and produce alternate contraction and rarefaction of sound-waves. Conversely they also produce electrical impulses when struck by a sound wave (Figure 1.2). If a single source (single crystal) were used, sound waves originating from it would resemble ripples in a pond. When multiple ripples from multiple elements originate, these coalesce to form a unidirectional wave front (Figure 1.3). Such a wave-front can be advanced in a sector by rotating the elements. This can be done either mechanically or by electric motors. The most popular transducers are electronic real time scanners that use the phased array principle. These transducers use multiple elements that are placed linearly and generate a linear wave front. The direction of the wave front can be altered by delaying sequential activation of the elements. The crystals can be placed in sets, one horizontal and other vertical to produce a biplane transducer or a single set can be rotated through 180 degrees as in a multi-plane transducer.

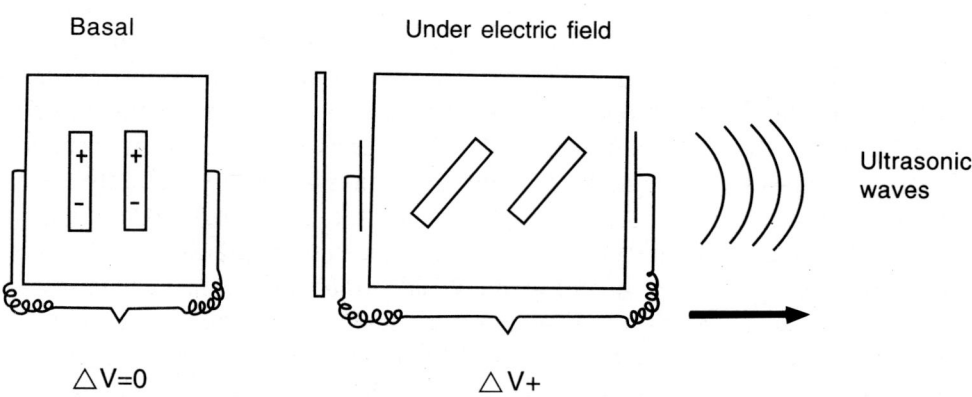

Figure 1.2. Principles of piezoelectric crystals:The crystal generates and receives sound waves using a principle called the piezoelectric (pressure electricity) effect, which was discovered by Pierre and Jacques Curie in 1880. In the probe, there are one or more quartz crystals called piezoelectric crystals. When an electric current is applied to these crystals (ΔV), they change shape rapidly. The rapid shape changes, or vibrations, of the crystals produce sound waves that travel outward. Conversely, when sound or pressure waves hit the crystals, they emit electrical currents. Therefore, the same crystals can be used to send and receive sound waves.

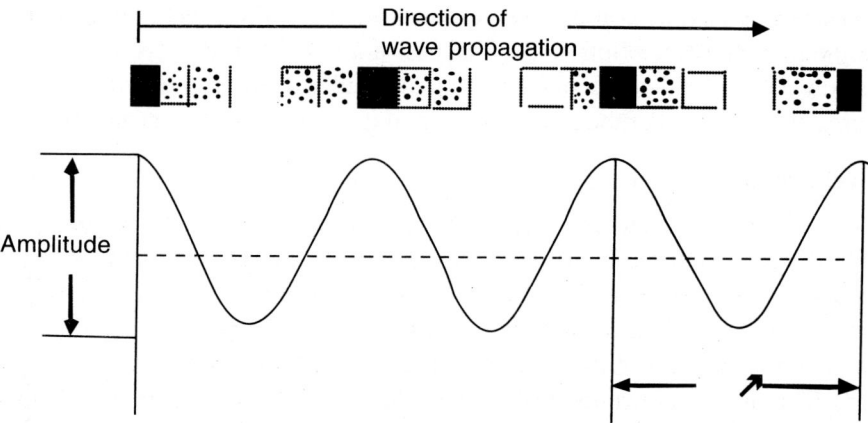

Figure 1.3. Ultrasound propagates through the medium in the shape of a sinuous curve. The permanent transmission of kinetic energy from one molecule to the next is performed in the form of a continuous wave which is referred to as sound wave. During this process, alternating phases of compression (pressure phase) and decompression (suction phase) can be observed in the matter. The wavelength ($\nearrow$) of a wave is the minimum distance in which a wave repeats itself. The frequency (f) of a wave is the number of waves per second.

Variables for real time imaging

A moving echo image on a television screen or monitor is made of frames. Usually projection of at least 30 frames/sec is required for eliminating the feel of a stationary image. Each frame is made up of two fields separated by a black line, not appreciated on the screen due to persistence of vision. Each field originates from one ultrasonic sweep. The time required for one sweep is determined by the pulse repetition frequency and sector angle. The rate of emission of ultrasonic waves, which occurs in brief intervals of time (1-2 micro sec), determines the pulse repetition frequency. Similarly the sweep time is also dependent on the sector angle, smaller the sector angle the more the time available for sweeping a given area. The sweep time in turn determines the number of lines in each sector. An image in ultrasound is made from multiple lines and its resolution depends upon the line density. The more the lines in one sector, the clearer would be the image. Since the velocity of ultrasound is 1540 m/sec, each line takes about 0.28 sec to refresh itself. Thus the smaller the sector angle, the higher would be the number of lines per degree, the more would be the line density and the higher would be the image resolution. To summarize, the variables that determine an image resolution on screen include line density, pulse repetition frequency, angle of the sweep and the frame rate.

M-mode and two-dimensional imaging

Apart from the emission of ultrasonic waves, the transducer becomes a receiver for the remaining (99%) period and receives the reflected wave. The reflected wave in turn hits the piezo-electric crystal to produce an electric current. If one knows the time delay then the distance of object can be computed and shown on an oscilloscope at a finite representative distance. The amplitude of the returning signal could be represented as a spike (A or amplitude mode) or in form of varying brightness (B-mode). Subsequent frames over a period of time could be represented on one of the axis to produce motion and called the M-mode or motion mode. The use of a B-mode image to create an exact image of an object in a field-sector and bringing in of subsequent frames with persistence of vision creates real time B-mode imaging or two dimensional echocardiography.

Doppler echocardiography

Doppler is a technique to detect the manner in which blood moves in the cardiovascular system. If the target is stationary, the frequency of the transmitted wave and the reflected waves are identical. If the target is moving towards the transducer, the received frequency is increased. If the target is moving away then the received frequency is reduced. The Doppler shift represents the difference between received and transmitted frequencies (Figure 1.4). The mathematical relation between the velocity of the target and Doppler frequency can be given by the following equation:

$$v = fd.c / 2ft (\cos \theta)$$

Where fd is the Doppler frequency, ft is the transmitted frequency,

and θ is the angle between path of travel and ultrasonic beam.

The best Doppler information is derived if the beam is parallel to the moving target with an angle between the beam and direction of the moving target not exceeding 20 degrees. Two types of Doppler application are used in clinical practice; continuous

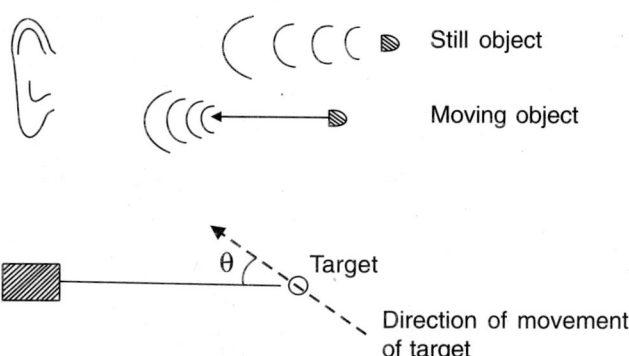

Figure 1.4. Doppler effect. Sound waves that are emitted from an object moving towards a reciever are compressed causing an increase in the frequency

and pulsed wave Doppler (Figure 1.5). In a continuous Doppler, a transducer is used with separate transmitting and receiving elements. This works continuously and hence there is no way to register the delay in receiving an incoming impulse, and thus the depth of an individual target or the location of a moving target cannot be estimated. On the contrary, in the pulsed-Doppler, the same transducer initially sends a burst of waves and then works as a receiver. By knowing the delay it is possible to compute the distance of a moving target or to obtain information from a given depth. However the major limitation of a pulsed Doppler is that it cannot measure velocities above a specific threshold. Since a finite time is required for transmitting a returning wave, a frequency higher than a specific threshold cannot be registered. This is called the aliasing velocity and the limit is called the Nyquist limit. Usually the Nyquist limit equals one-half pulse repetition frequency.

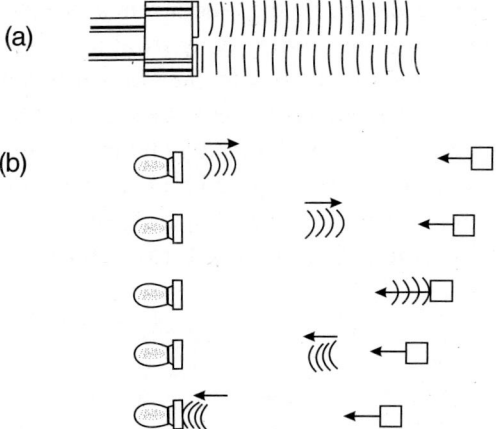

Figure 1.5. Principles of continuous wave(CW) and pulsed wave(PW) Doppler. The CW transducer **(a)** emits and recieves simultaneously through two different crystals. The PW Doppler transducer **(b)** emits short pulses of ultrasound waves, the distance of interrogation is determined by the reception delay; the speed of the target is calculated by the difference between emitted and received frequencies.

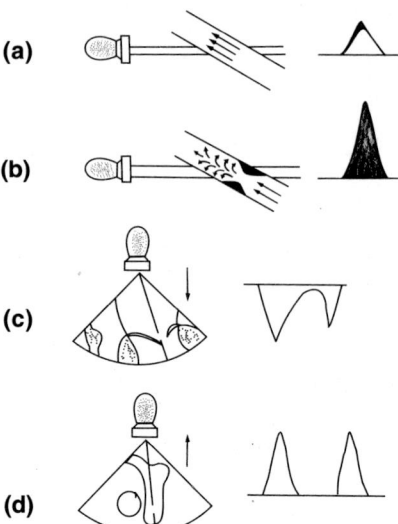

Figure 1.6. Types of blood flow seen on spectral Doppler display. **(a)** shows laminar flow, **(b)** turbulent flow, **(c)** blood flow moving away from transducer (for transmitral flow) and **(d)** flow towards transducer (flow in pulmonary artery).

The Doppler information is usually displayed graphically against time and is called the spectral Doppler. The spectral Doppler is useful for computing velocity and pressure gradients, valve orifice areas and blood flow (Figure 1.6). Pulsed Doppler information from a given field sector can be represented at multiple points at multiple depths with different colours, each colour denoting a particular frequency. This is called the colour Doppler and forms the basis of colour-flow imaging. The Doppler flow is usually superimposed on the two-dimensional cardiac image. The physiologic motion of moving flow determines the direction; traditionally the colour red is assigned to motion towards the transducer and the colour blue for motion away from the transducer with multiple shades of green and yellow for intermediate velocities in a turbulent flow. Since colour Doppler uses the concept of pulsed-Doppler, higher velocities are not properly represented and result in aliasing. As the image aliases the colour changes from blue to red and vice-versa. Another limitation is the higher time required for colour-flow imaging, this reduces the frame rate. Therefore for optimizing the image resolution, the sector angle and region of interrogation for the colour-Doppler needs to be much smaller than the actual 2-D image.

Chapter 2

CARDIAC ASSESSMENT

STANDARD IMAGING PROCEDURES

Introduction

Trans-oesophageal echocardiography (TOE) is an accepted monitoring tool inside the cardiac operation theatre. Although, its use was first described in 1980, it did not become commonplace until high-frequency transducers and colour Doppler imaging became available in the mid-1980s. In India, it became available only in the late 1990s. The improvement in the quality of the acoustic image has enabled anaesthesiologists and surgeons to use TOE intraoperatively to diagnose myocardial ischaemia, confirm the adequacy of valve and other surgical repairs, determine the cause of haemodynamic disorders and other intraoperative complications, and provide diagnostic information that could not be obtained preoperatively. Indeed, the use of TOE has facilitated the prevention and early treatment of perioperative complications. The advantages of TOE over conventional transthoracic echocardiography include better acoustic images and continuation of monitoring even when the chest is open during the surgery.

Anaesthesiologists using the TOE must have adequate knowledge of cardiac anatomy and physiology and of ultrasound technology. In addition, he must acquire the essential technical skills for the use of TOE.

Technique of TOE examination

Initially, a monoplane probe was used for TOE. With advances in ultrasound technology, a biplane probe was introduced in the early 1990s and was soon replaced by the omniplane (multiplane) probe.[1] Perioperatively TOE is performed in the supine position in an anaesthetised and intubated or sedated or unconscious patient in the operation theatre or intensive care unit.

It should be ensured before the insertion of the probe that it has been disinfected and that the control wheels are working and unlocked. Basically, the probe is a gastroscope equipped with ultrasound instead of fibreoptic technology. The phased-array transducer is integrated into the flexible tip of the probe that has a diameter of 10-15 mm and length of 20-45 mm. The shaft of the probe has a diameter of 9-10 mm and is about 100 cm long. The position of the flexible tip can be varied by rotation of the two steering wheels at the handle of the probe. The bigger wheel helps anteflexion or retroflexion, whereas the smaller wheel provides left and right lateral flexion. The wheels and therefore, the tip of the probe can be locked in an optimum position for monitoring purposes.

Probe insertion

The ultrasound machine is positioned behind the patient's head at the left side. The insertion of the probe must be smooth and no force should be applied. The stomach should be aspirated and gastric tube removed before insertion of the probe. This helps to remove the gastric secretions as well as air that might degrade the quality of the image. The assistant holds the handle of the probe and the operator opens the mouth and lifts the jaw of the patient with the left hand and with the right hand he gently introduces the tip (that is lubricated with lignocaine jelly) into the oropharynx and oesophagus. A slight degree of anteflexion of the tip may be required for the entry into the oesophagus. The biting block should be used in all patients (except those who are edentulous) so that injury to the probe by teeth is prevented during the movement of the probe. Some operators use the index and middle finger of the left hand to guide the probe through the pharynx. This blind technique of probe insertion is almost always successful but increased jaw and chin lift or slight rotation of the head may be required. Very rarely, a laryngoscope may be necessary to facilitate the insertion. The probe is advanced approximately 30 cm from the teeth and is connected to the console. A hyperinflated tracheal cuff of the endotracheal tube may offer resistance high in the oesophagus, while stenosis or stricture of the hiatus may do so lower down in the oesophagus. It must be remembered that force should not be applied to overcome resistance at any stage during the probe insertion.

Manipulation of the probe

With the omniplane probe the steering of the ultrasound beam is automated, usually by pressing a knob on the handle. However, some manually controlled movement of the probe will be necessary to obtain the optimum image in a given patient. Transverse plane imaging (usually 0° angle on the multiplane probe) usually provides transverse or horizontal sections of the heart, whereas longitudinal plane imaging gives longitudinal or vertical sections. During a longitudinal plane examination, clockwise or anticlockwise rotation of the probe can shift the vertical plane to the right or left. With clockwise rotation, the vertical plane shifts to the right so that structures on the right such as superior vena cava and right pulmonary veins are visualised, whereas anticlockwise rotation helps to visualise structures on the left such as left atrial appendage and the left pulmonary veins. Thus, the probe requires up and down movement in order to obtain transverse sections of the heart at various levels and rotation of the probe to obtain vertical sections. With the help of the knob on the handle and the manual movement of the probe, a comprehensive examination of various cardiac structures can be performed using the multiplane probe.

A small semicircular icon on the screen displays the position of the imaging plane between 0° and 180°. The transducer scanning sector is fan shaped, and appears as such on the monitor screen. The narrowest portion of the fan lies closest to the transducer (posterior aspect). The wide portion of the fan represents the anterior aspect of the image.

In this chapter, standard views obtained during TOE examination are illustrated.

1. Seward JB, Khanderia BK, Freeman WK, et al: Multiplane transesophageal echocardiography: image orientation, examination technique, anatomic correlations, and clinical applications. *Mayo Clin Proc* 1993;68:523-5.

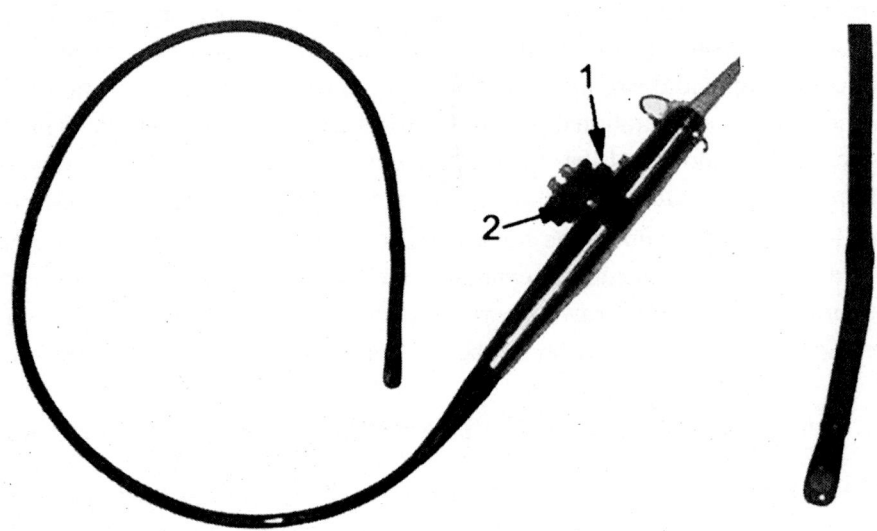

Figure 2.1. Adult TOE Probe. The probe is a 100-cm modified gastroscope. There are two control knobs on the handle of the probe. The larger inner knob (arrow 1) controls anterior and posterior flexion and the smaller outer knob (arrow 2) controls leftward and rightward angulation.

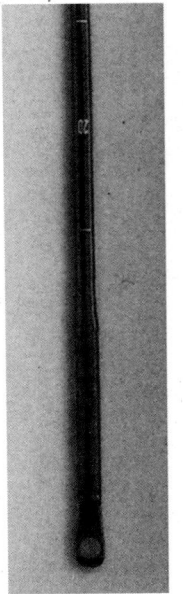
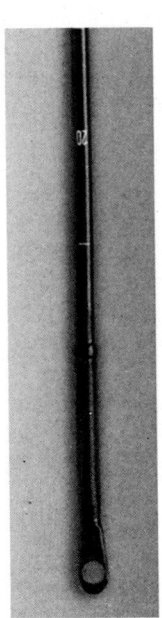
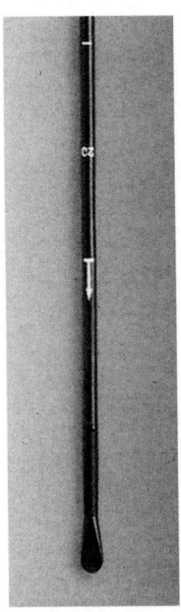

Figure 2.2. Different types of probes for performing trans-oesophageal echocardiography. From left to right: Omniplane II probe (4-7 MHz frequency) Omniplane III probe (2-7 MHz frequency range that provides the bandwidth for harmonic imaging and contrast research applications), and Omniplane paediatric probe.

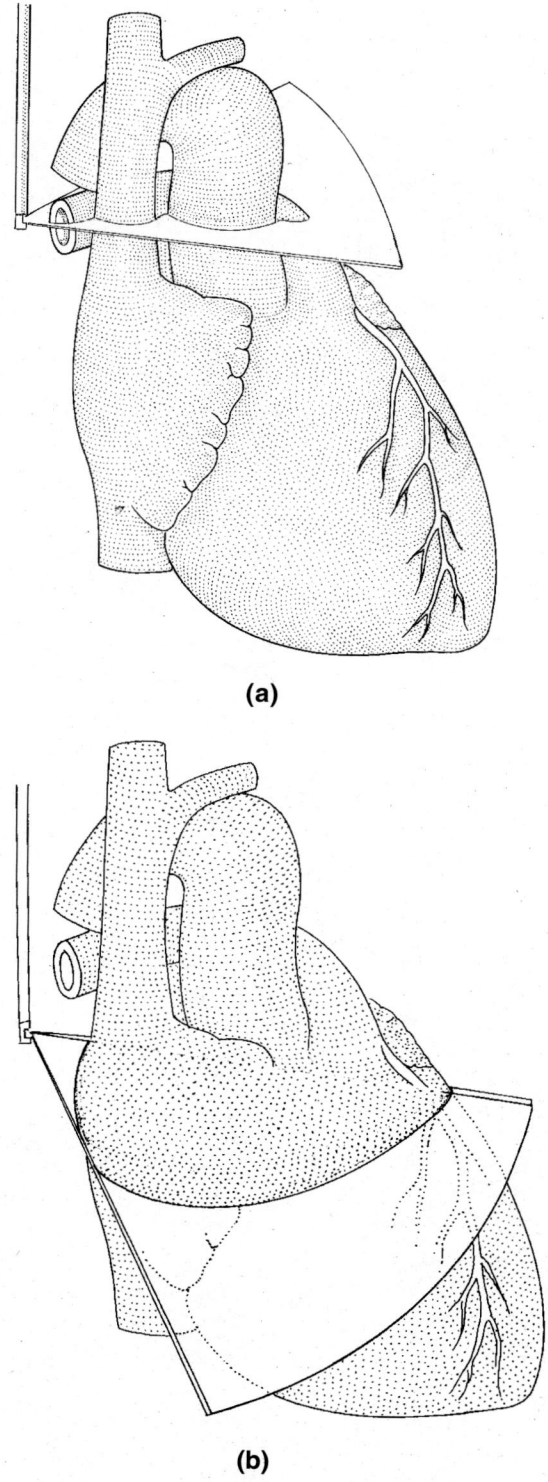

(a)

(b)

Figure 2.3 (a) Diagrammatic representation of ultrasound beam in upper oesophageal view, **(b)** Diagrammatic representation of ultrasound beam in mid-oesophageal view.

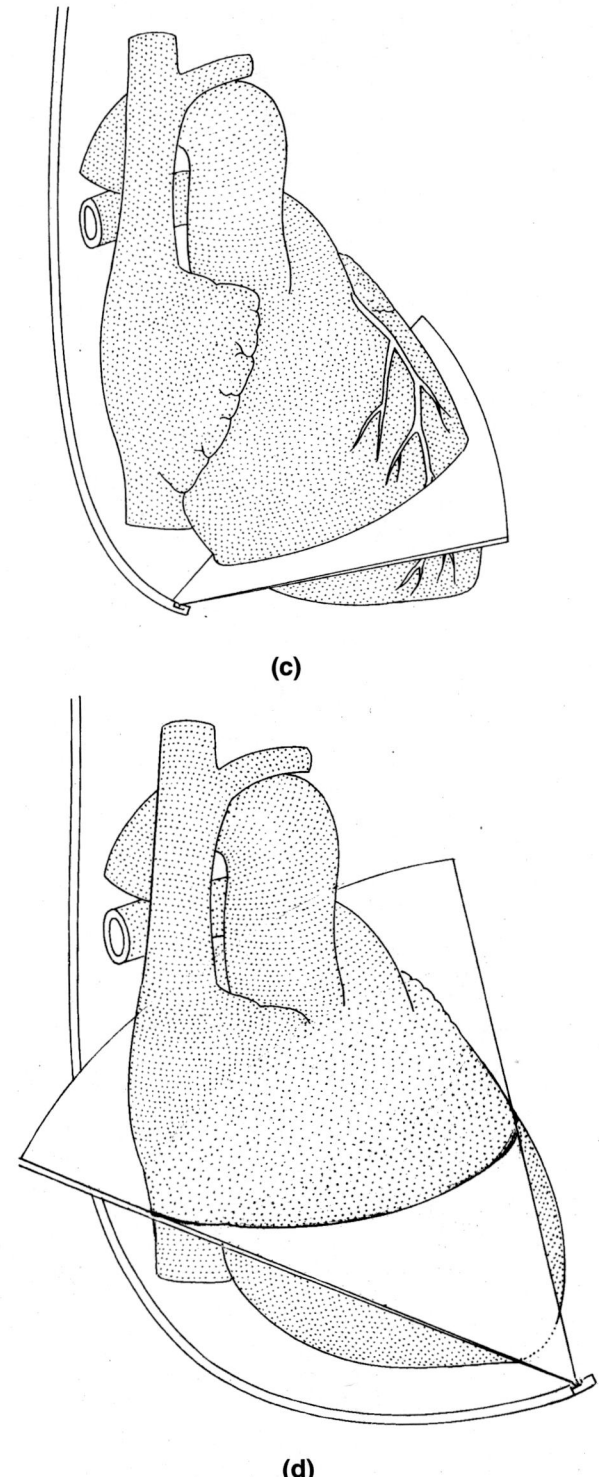

(c)

(d)

Figure 2.3 (c) Diagrammatic representation of ultrasound beam in proximal transgastric view, **(d)** Diagrammatic representation of ultrasound beam in deep transgastric view.

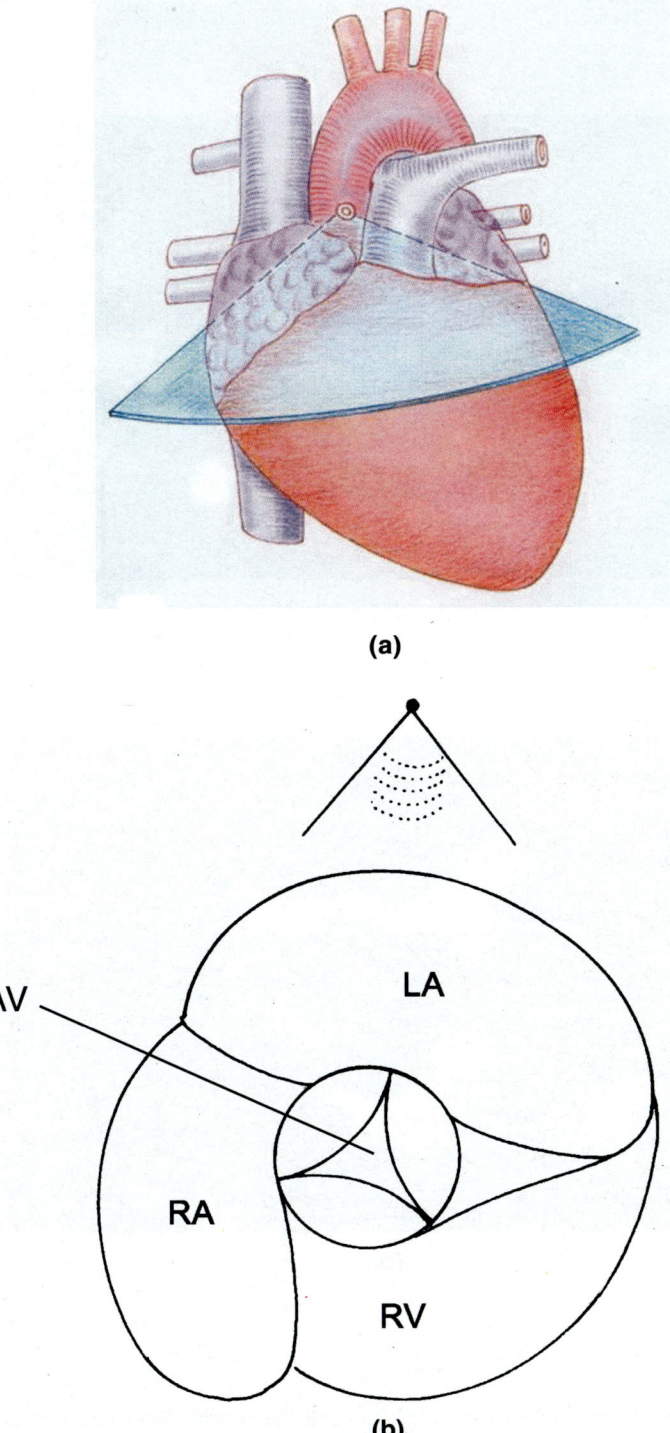

(a)

(b)

Figure 2.4. Upper oesophageal view (40-60°).
(a & b) Diagrammatic representation of ultrasound beam and resultant image. (LA: left atrium, RA: right atrium, RV: right ventricle, AV: aortic valve)

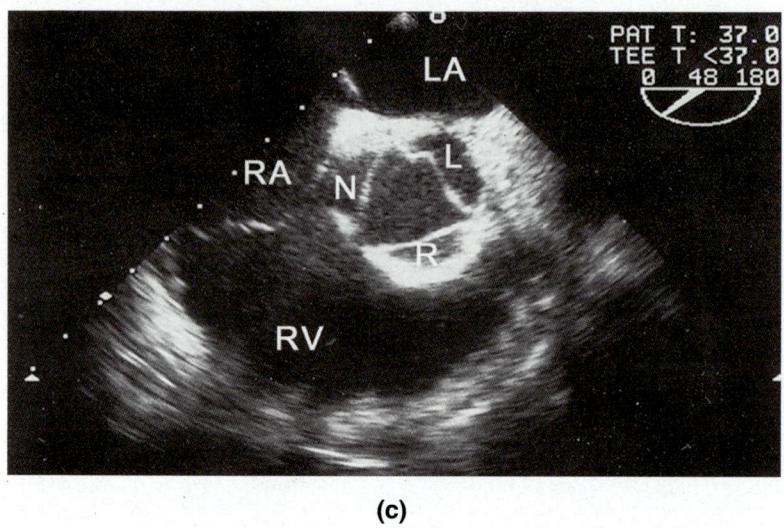

(c)

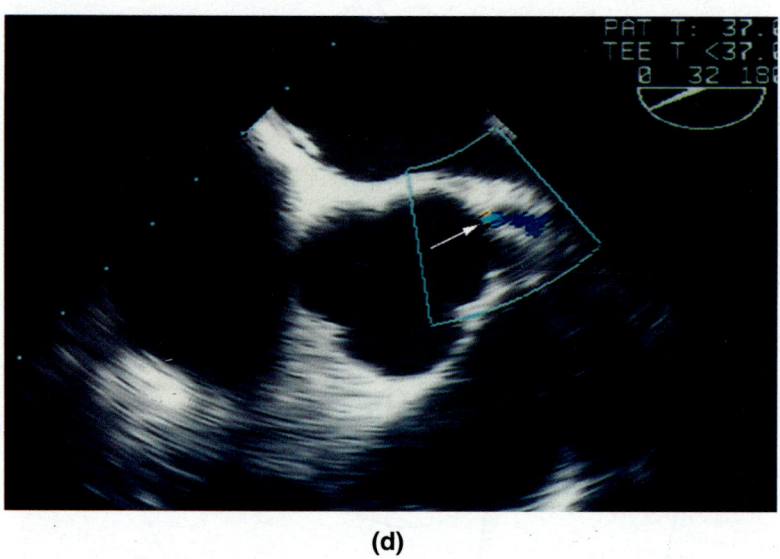

(d)

Figure 2.4 (c) This is an important view that images the aortic valve in short axis. The left coronary cusp (L) is on the right side, the right coronary cusp (R) is at the bottom and the noncoronary cusp (N) lies on the left. **(d)** The left main coronary artery can be seen originating at this level (arrow) and can be followed further till its bifurcation. (LA: left atrium, RA: right atrium, RV: right ventricle)

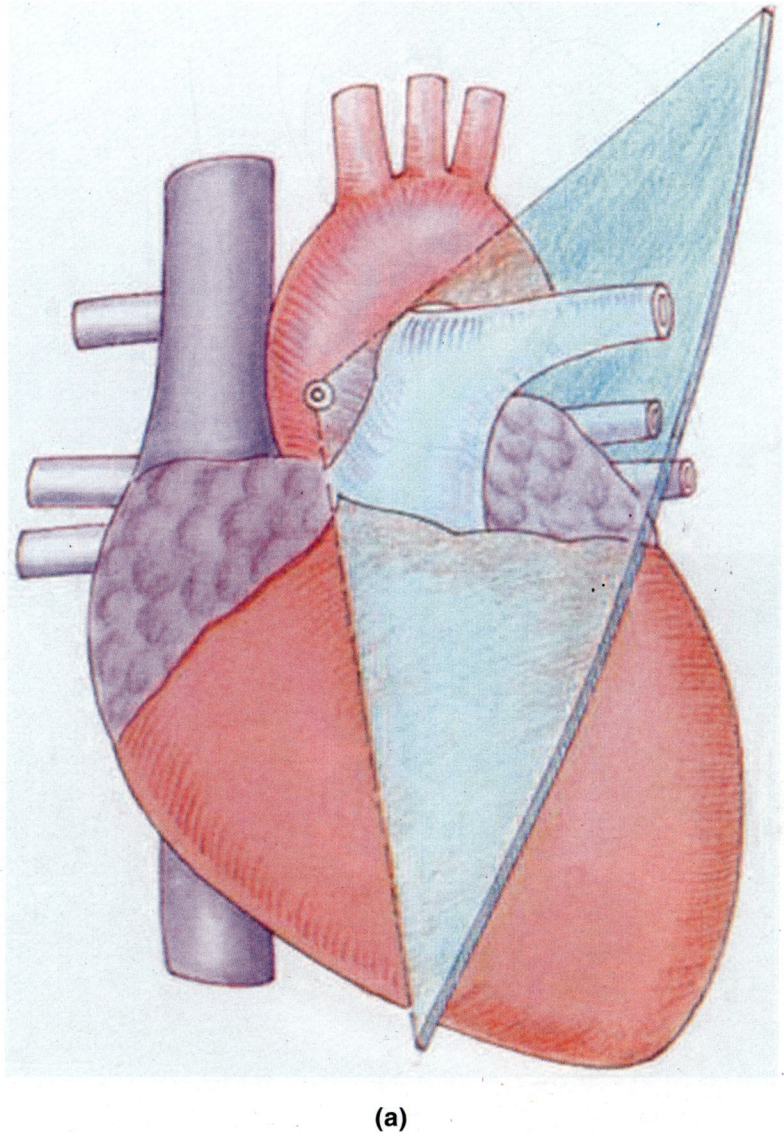

(a)

Figure 2.5. Upper oesophageal view (60-100°).
(a) Diagrammatic representation of ultrasound beam.

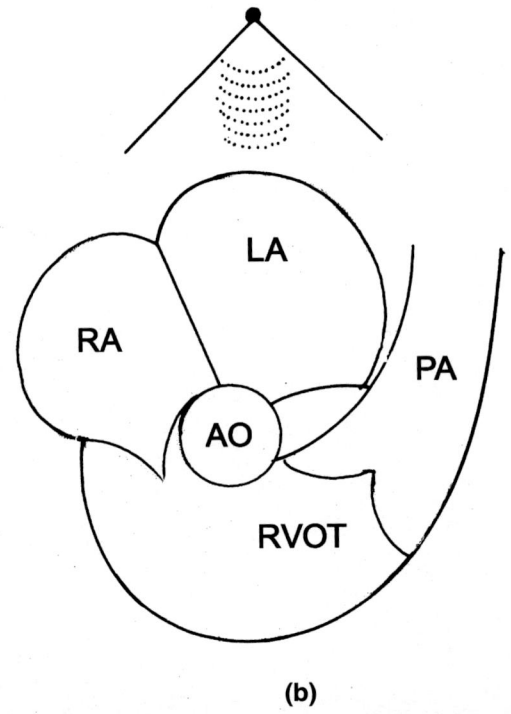

(b)

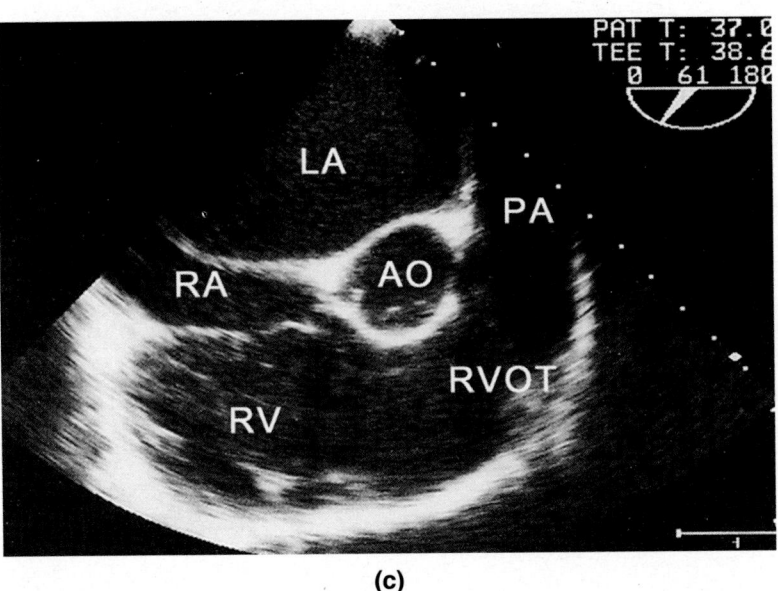

(c)

Figure 2.5 (b) Diagrammatic representation of ultrasound image. **(c)** The transverse section of the aorta remains in the middle and left atrium lies at the top of the screen, while from left to right, the right atrium, tricuspid valve, right ventricle, pulmonary valve, and the main pulmonary artery are visualised as they circle around the aorta. The view is useful for the evaluation of the right ventricular outflow tract, especially in the congenital lesions involving the right ventricle and pulmonary artery. (LA: left atrium, RA: right atrium, AO: aorta, RVOT: right ventricular outflow tract, PA: pulmonary artery)

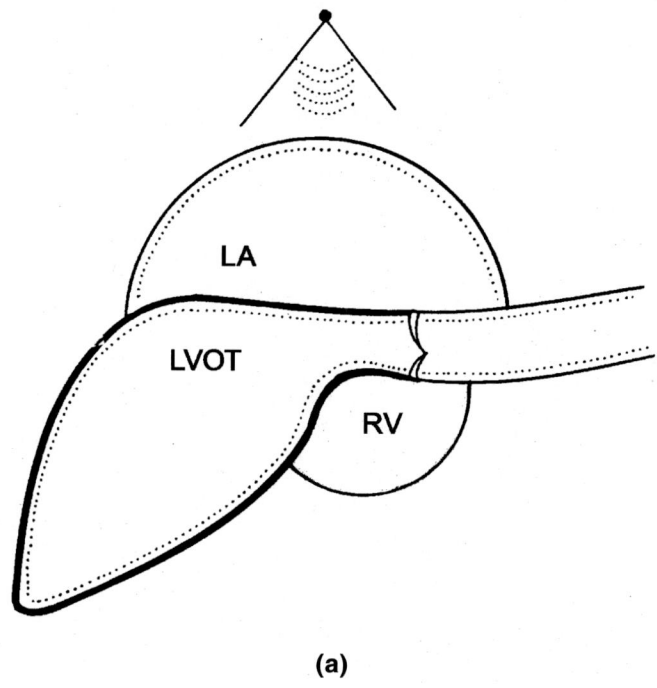

(a)

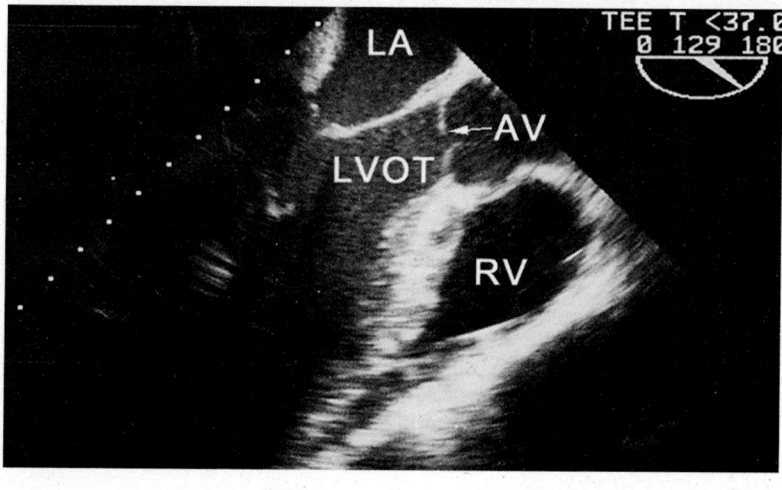

(b)

Figure 2.6. Upper oesophageal view (110-130º).
(a) Diagrammatic representation of ultrasound image. **(b)** The imaging plane beyond 110º
displays the distal part of the left ventricular outflow tract, the aortic valve and ascending
aorta in the longitudinal axis. (LA: left atrium, LVOT: left ventricular outflow tract, AV:
aortic valve, RV: right ventricle)

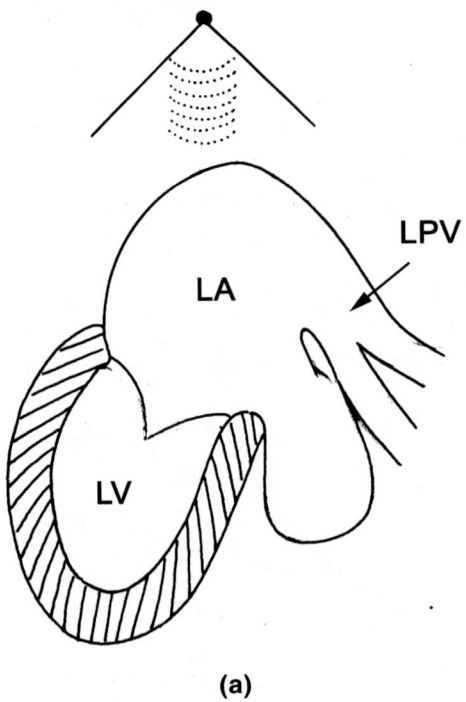

(a)

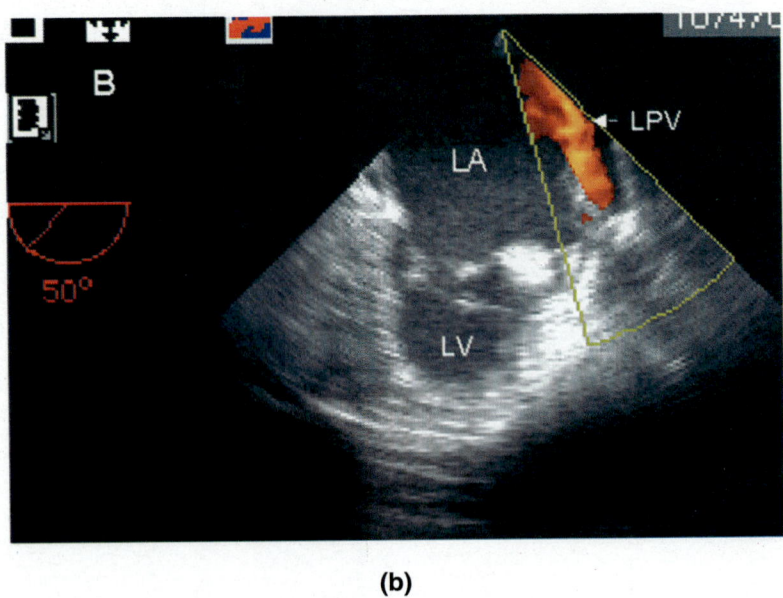

(b)

Figure 2.7. Left pulmonary vein view (20-40°).
(a) Diagrammatic representation of ultrasound image, **(b)** At 0-30° imaging plane, the left pulmonary vein can be visualised above the left atrial appendage. The left upper pulmonary vein has a more vertical and the lower one has a more horizontal course. This view can be used for Doppler interrogation of the pulmonary veins. (LA: left atrium, LV: left ventricle, LPV: left upper pulmonary vein)

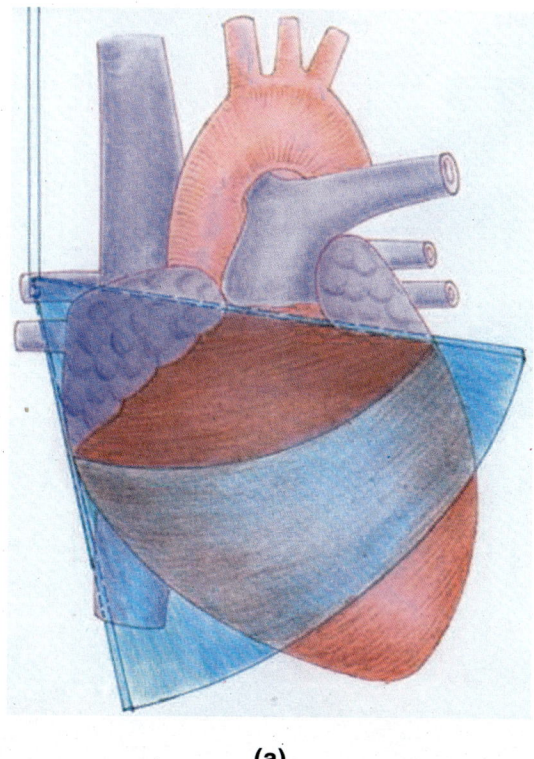

(a)

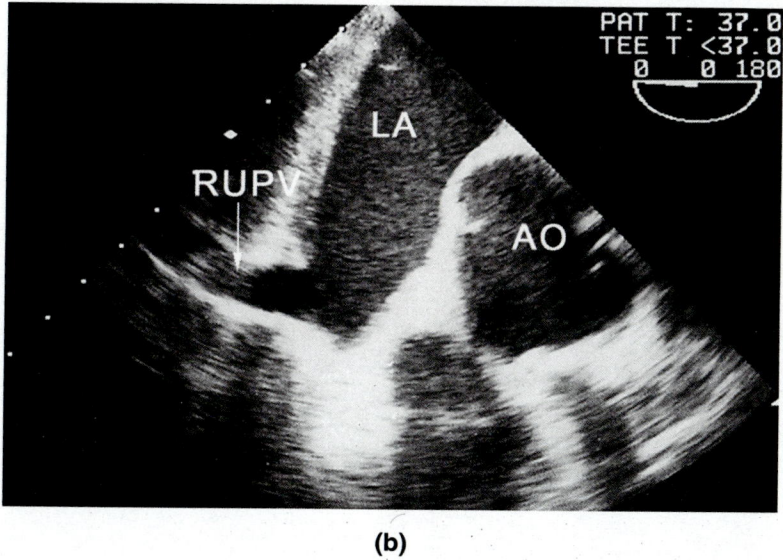

(b)

Figure 2.8. Right pulmonary vein view (0°).
(a) Diagrammatic representation of ultrasound beam. **(b)** The right upper and lower pulmonary veins can be visualised on the left of the sector at 0° as they enter the left atrium from the right. Rotation of the imaging plane to facilitate the best view is required. (RUPV: right upper pulmonary vein, LA: left atrium, AO: aorta)

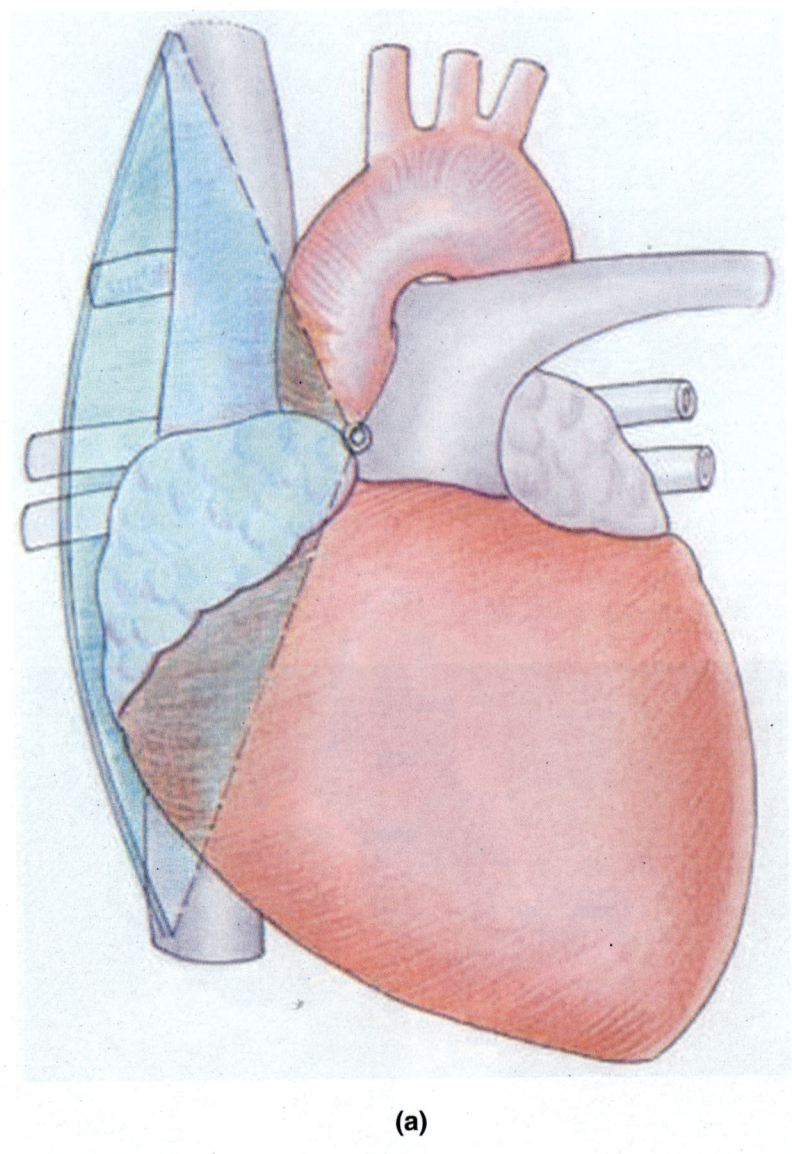

(a)

Figure 2.9. Bicaval view (120-130°).
(a) Diagrammatic representation of ultrasound beam.

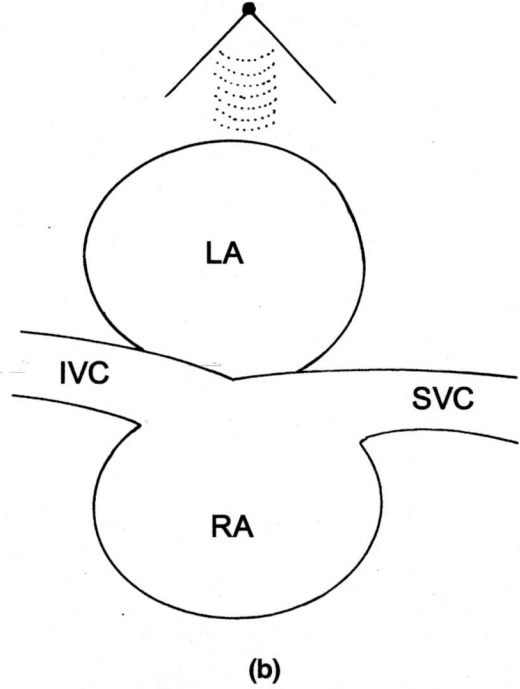

(b)

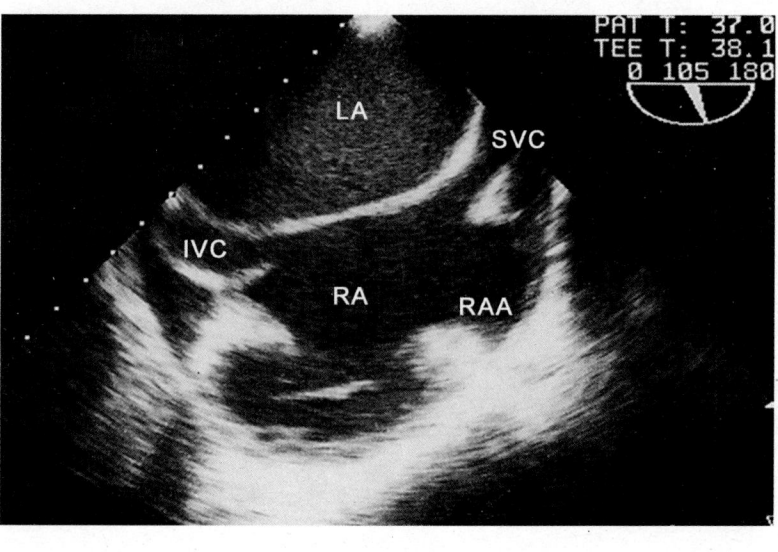

(c)

Figure 2.9 (b) Diagrammatic representation of ultrasound image. **(c)** This is an extremely important view for evaluating the anatomy of the inter-atrial septum. Inferior vena cava is seen on the left, superior vena cava on the right connected by the inter-atrial septum. Left atrium lies at the top. The TOE probe needs to be rotated clockwise to obtain this view. (LA: left atrium, IVC: inferior vena cava, SVC: superior vena cava, RA: right atrium, RAA: right atrial appendage)

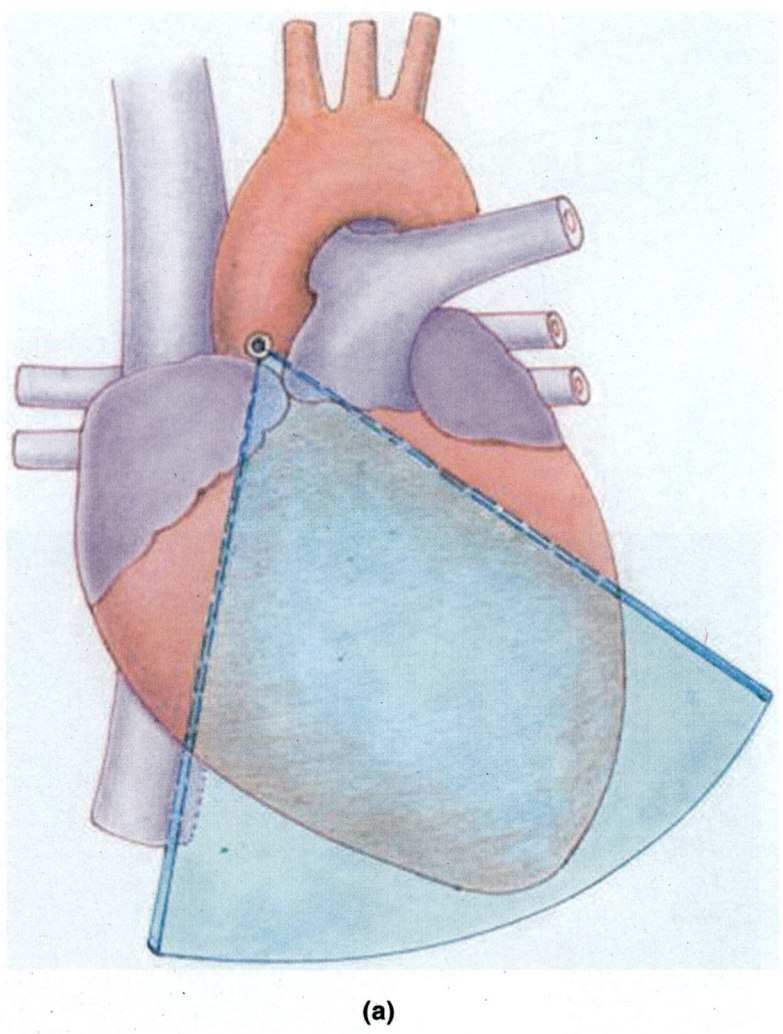

(a)

Figure. 2.10. Four chamber view (0º).
(a) Diagrammatic representation of ultrasound beam.

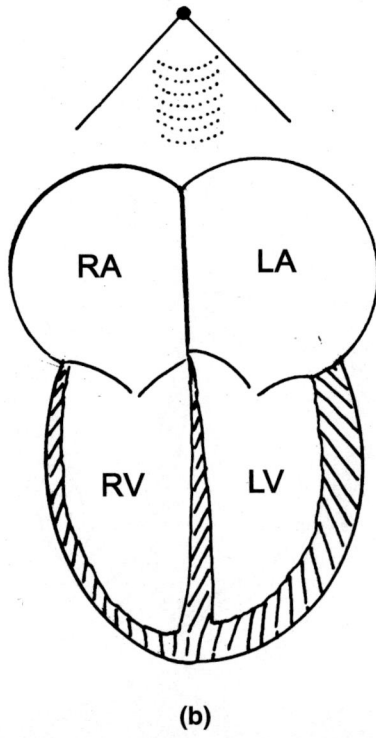

(b)

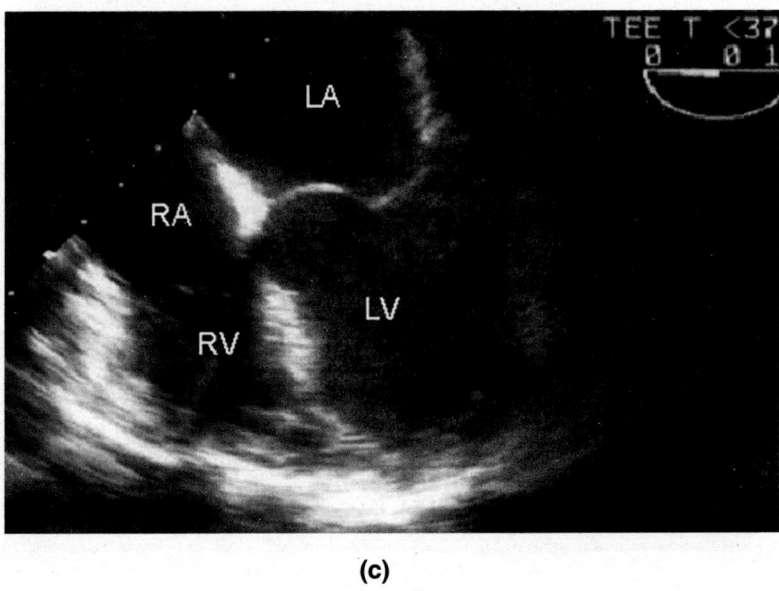

(c)

Figure. 2.10 (b) Diagrammatic representation of ultrasound image. **(c)** This is the standard four chamber view with both atria and both ventricles. The lateral free walls of both ventricles and the posterior portion of the inter-ventricular septum are seen. The mitral valve is close to the transducer and can be examined in detail.

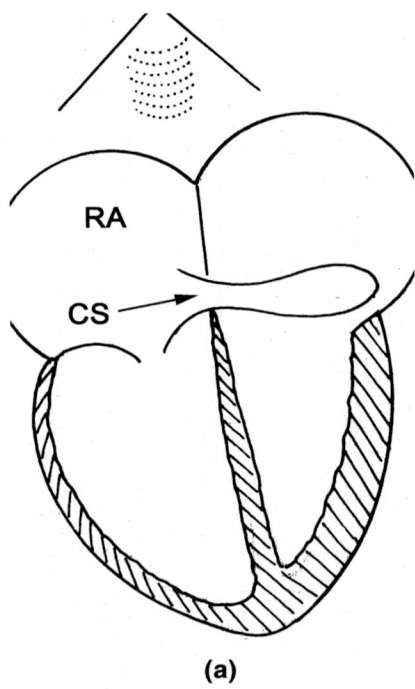

(a)

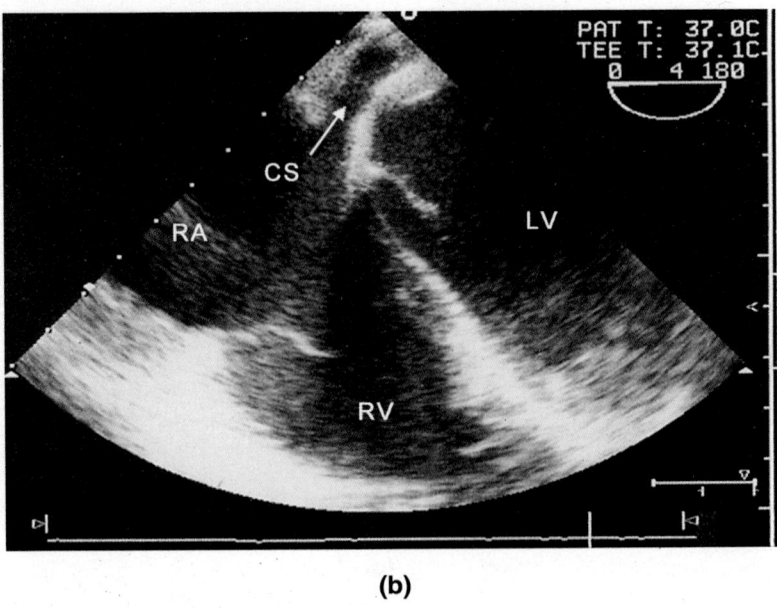

(b)

Figure 2.11. Four chamber view (0º).

(a) Diagrammatic representation of the coronary sinus. **(b)** By advancing the probe a little further (1 cm), after obtaining four chamber view, the coronary sinus can be profiled opening into the right atrium. (LA: left atrium, RA: right atrium, RV: right ventricle, LV: left ventricle, CS: coronary sinus)

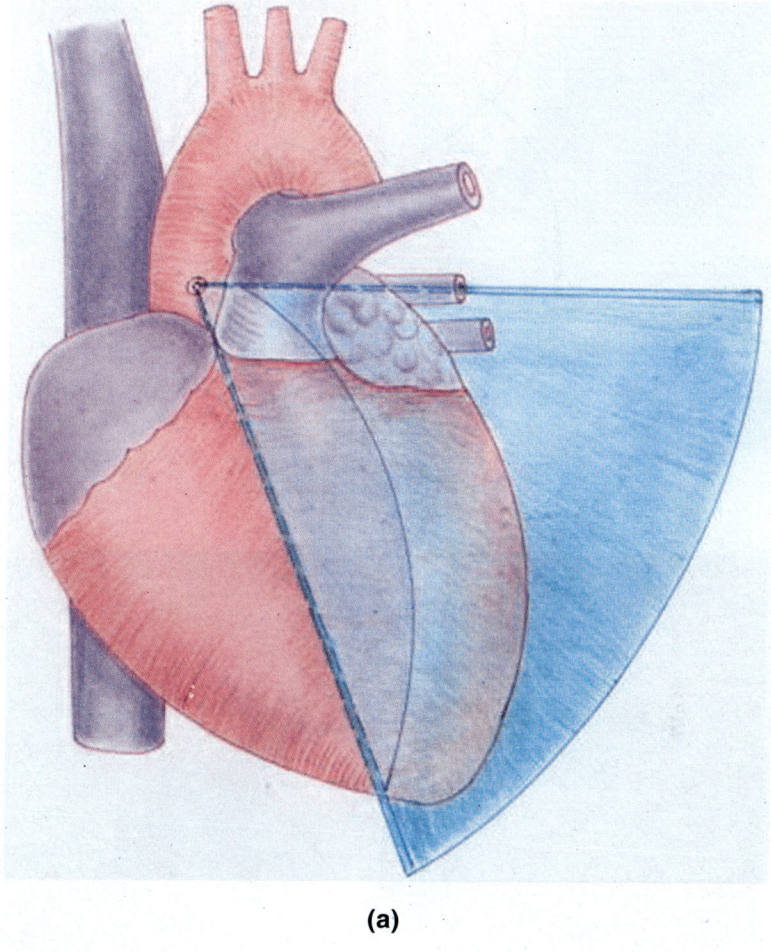

(a)

Figure 2.12. Two chamber view (90°).
(a) Diagrammatic representation of ultrasound beam.

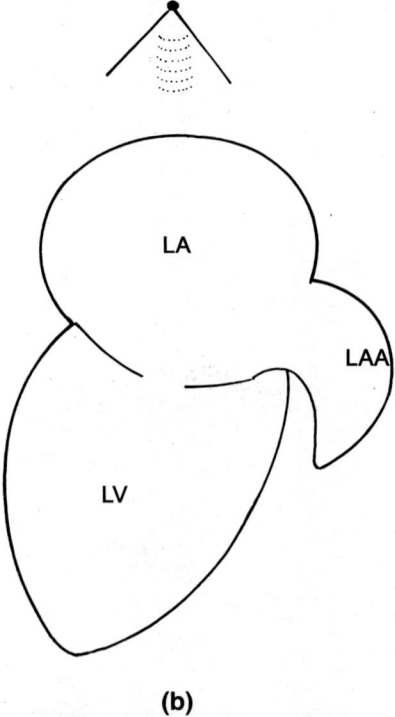

(b)

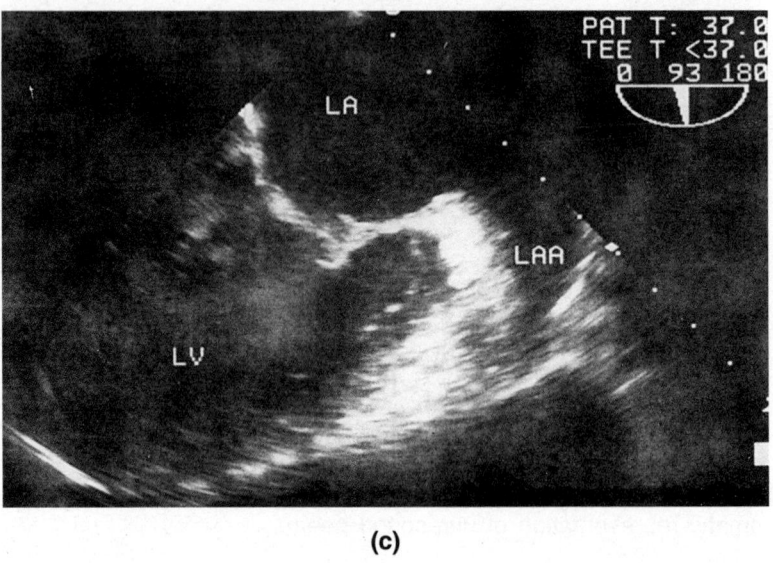

(c)

Figure 2.12 (b) Diagrammatic representation of ultrasound image. **(c)** By rotating the plane to 90°, the two chamber view with the left atrium at the top and the left ventricle below is obtained. The view helps to examine the mitral valve and the left ventricular wall motion abnormality of the inferior wall (left of the sector) and anterior wall (right of the sector). The left atrial appendage can also be seen. (LA: left atrium, LV: left ventricle, LAA: left atrial appendage)

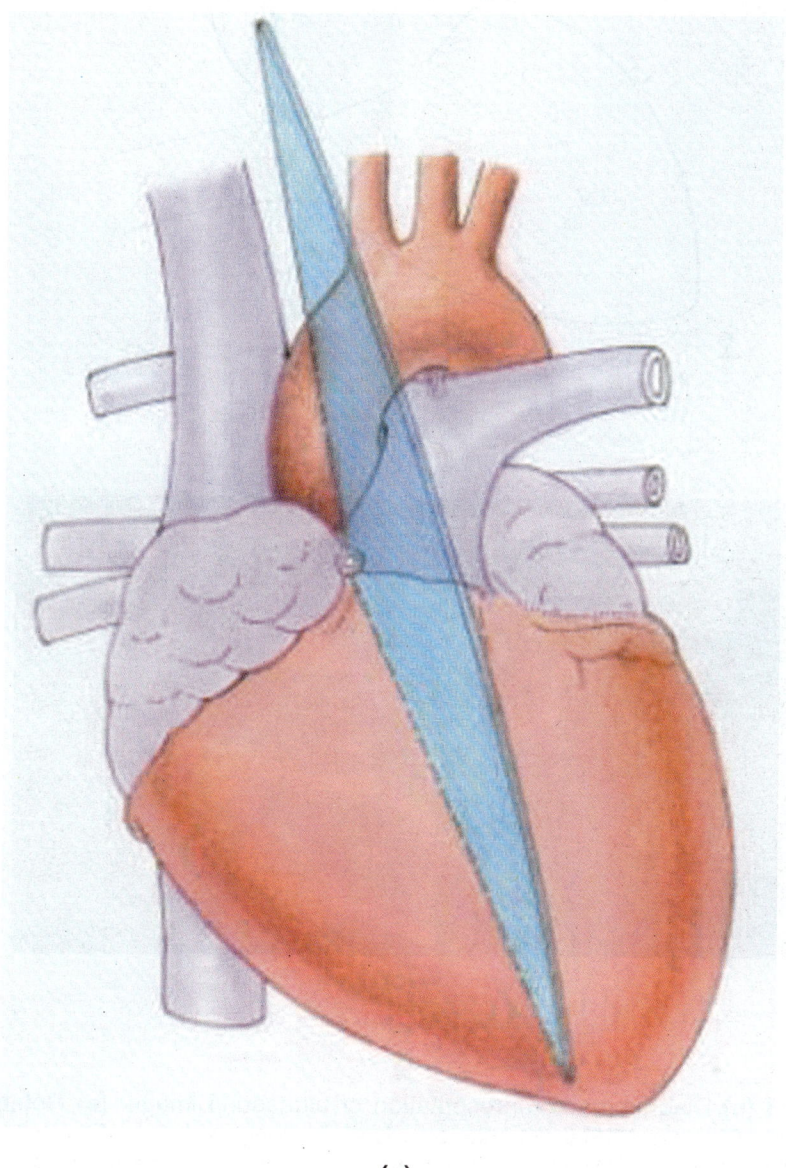

(a)

Figure 2.13. Three chamber view (130-150°).
(a) Diagrammatic representation of ultrasound beam.

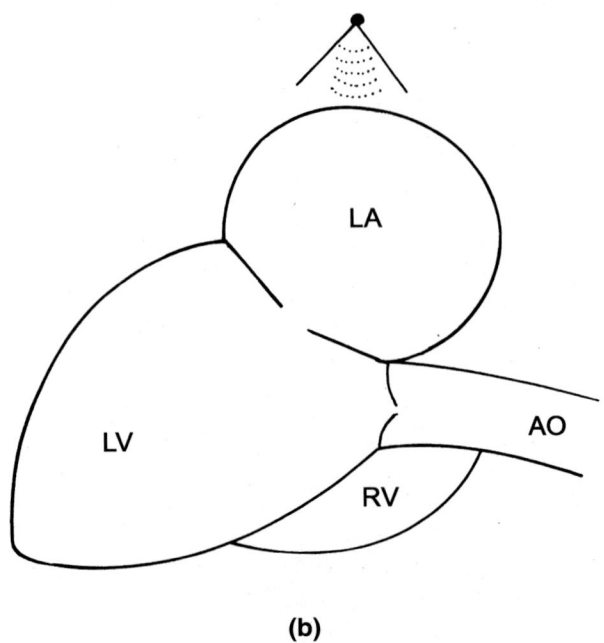

(b)

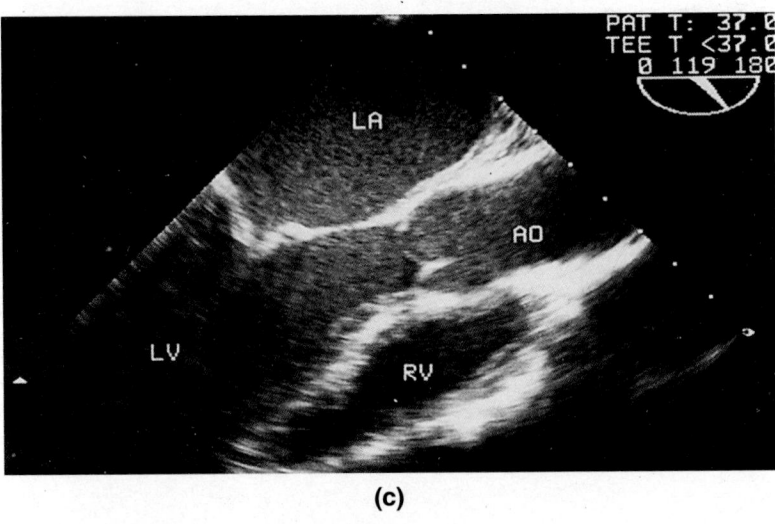

(c)

Figure 2.13 (b) Diagrammatic representation of ultrasound image. **(c)** Rotation of the plane to 130-150° shows the three chamber view. The long axis view of the left atrium, left ventricular outflow, aortic valve and a part of the ascending aorta is obtained. The noncoronary (top) and right coronary cusps of the aortic valve are visible. Postero-basal to postero-lateral wall forms the left sided and the anterior septum the right sided boundary of the left ventricle in this view. This view helps to examine aortic and mitral valves and subaortic ventricular septal defect. (LA: left atrium, LV: left ventricle, RV: right ventricle, AO: aorta)

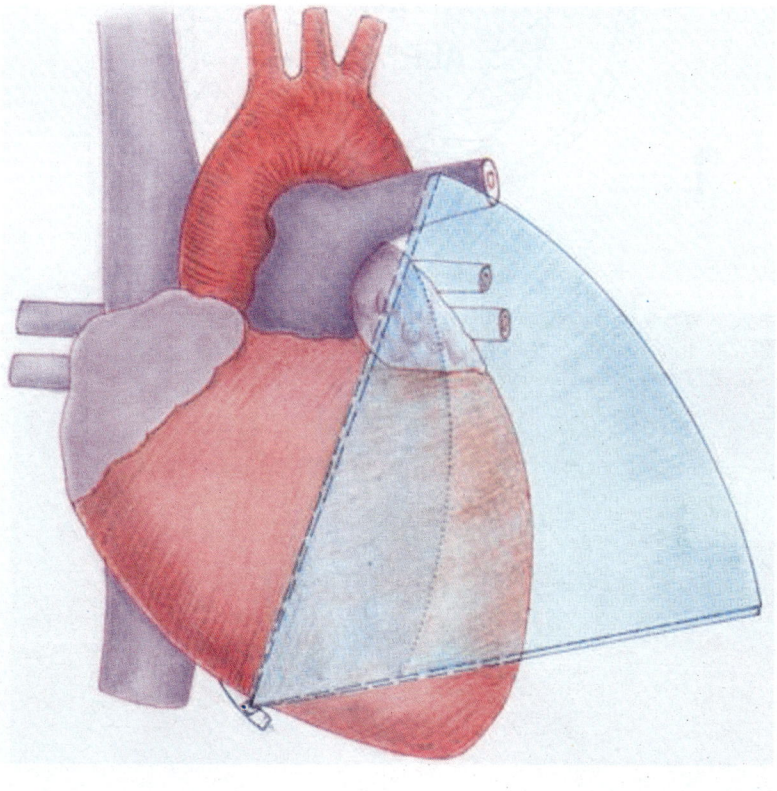

(a)

Figure 2.14. Transgastric short axis view of the left ventricle.
(a) Diagrammatic representation of ultrasound beam.

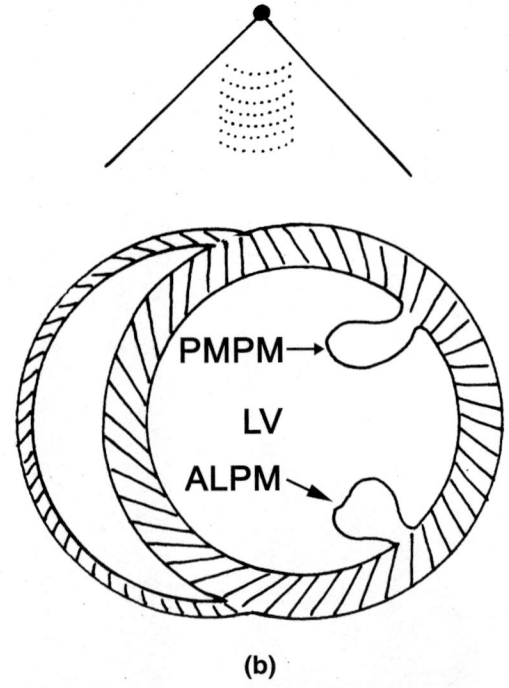

(b)

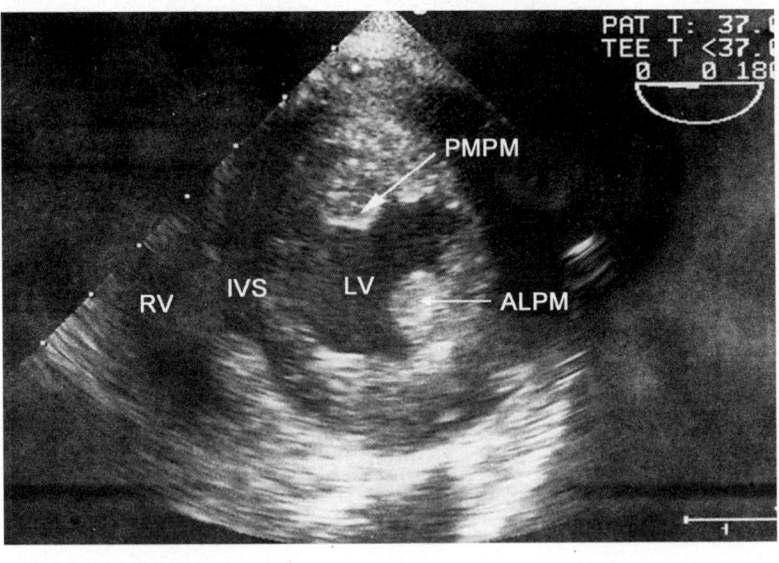

(c)

Figure 2.14 (b) Diagrammatic representation of short axis view of the left ventricle at mid papillary level. **(c)** The standard short axis view of the left ventricle at mid-papillary muscle level is the most commonly employed view. The inferior left ventricular wall lies at the top of the section, close to the transducer, and the anterior wall at the bottom. The interventricular septum is located on the left of the image and the lateral wall is seen on the right side. (PMPM: posteromedial papillary muscle, ALPM: anterolateral papillary muscle, IVS: interventricular septum, LV: left ventricle, RV: right ventricle)

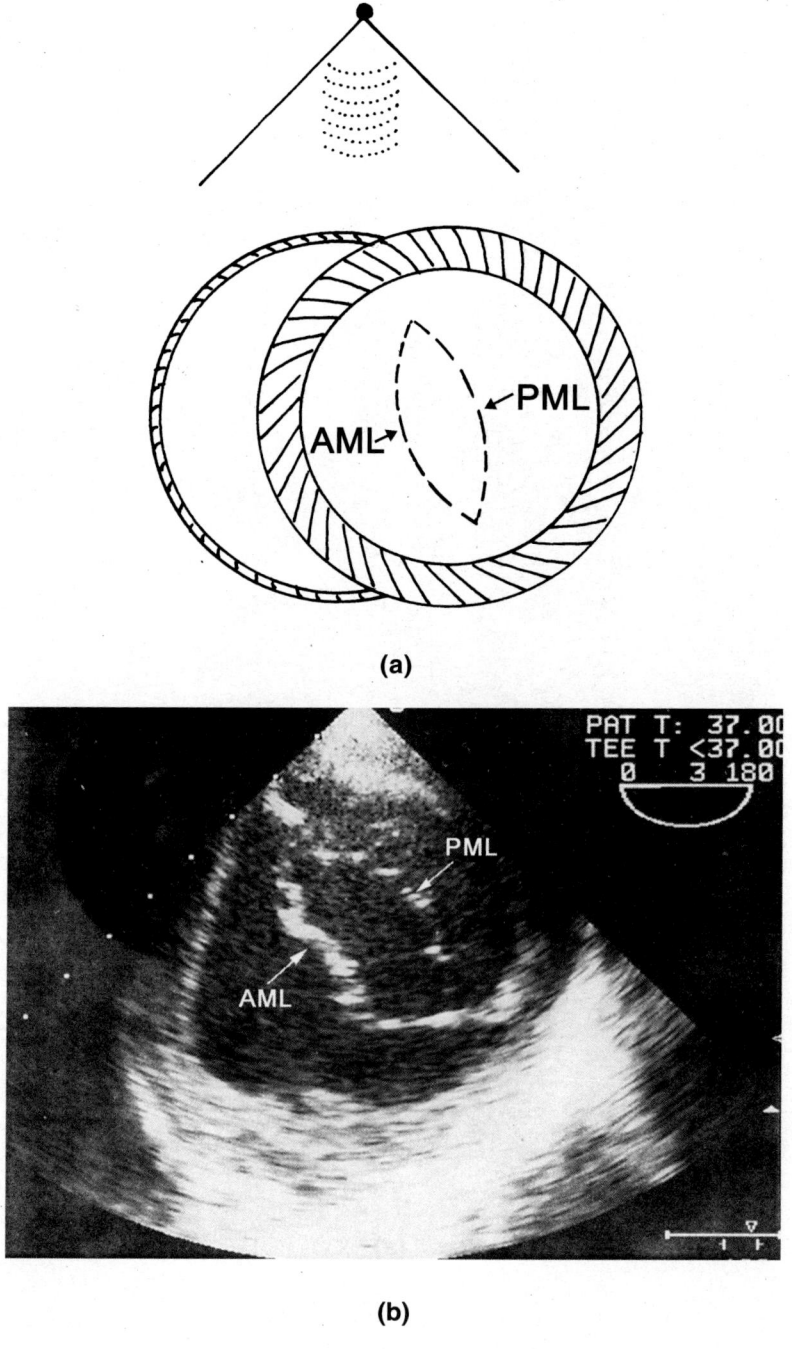

Figure 2.15 (a) Diagrammatic representation of basal short axis view of the left ventricle. **(b)** Basal short axis view of the left ventricle. (AML: anterior mitral leaflet, PML: posterior mitral leaflet)

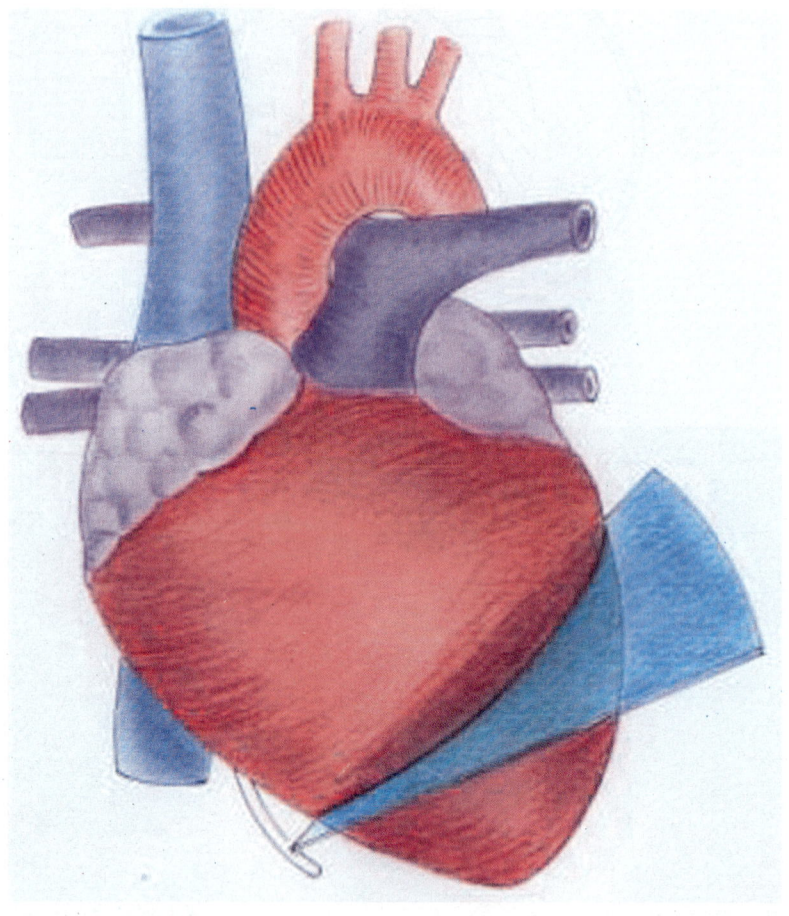

(a)

Figure 2.16. Apical short axis view of the left ventricle.
(a) Diagrammatic representation of the ultrasound beam.

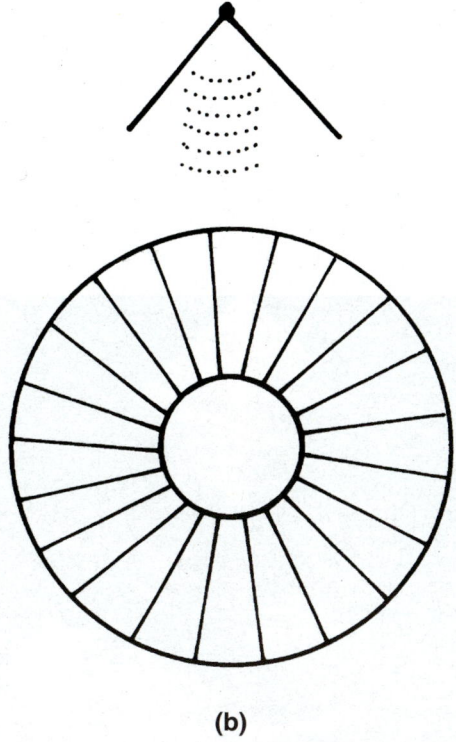

(b)

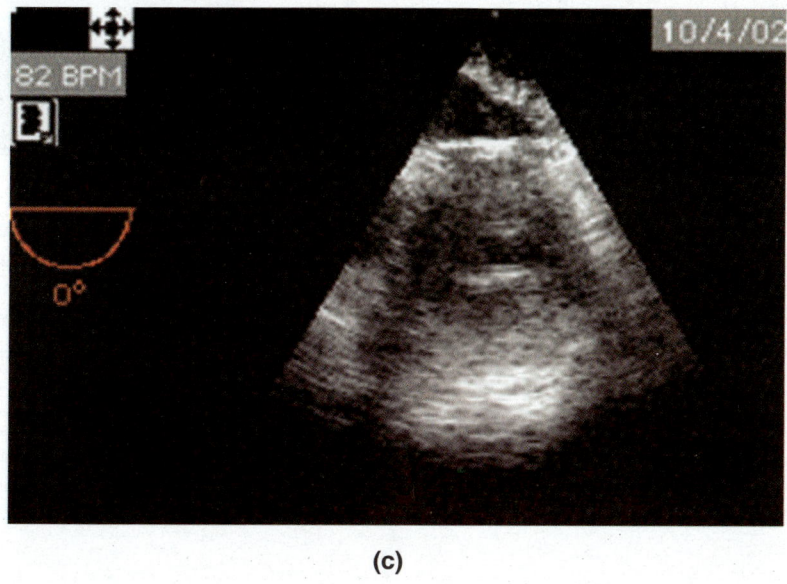

(c)

Figure 2.16 (b) Diagrammatic representation of ultrasound image. **(c)** By advancing the probe little further after obtaining mid-papillary view, this view can be obtained. Generally, it is difficult to obtain a clear image.

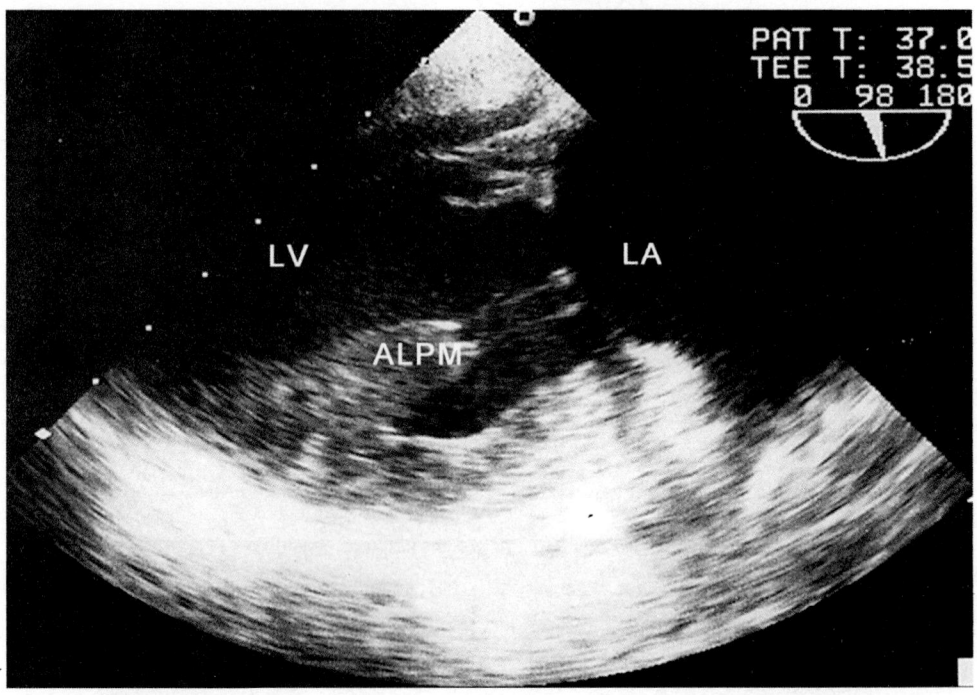

Figure 2.17. Long axis view of the left ventricle and left atrium. This view is derived from the short axis view of the left ventricle by rotating the imaging plane from 0-90⁰ and beyond. At 90 degrees, the long axis view of the left atrium, mitral valve, two papillary muscles and the left ventricle are obtained. The anterior wall of the left ventricle is at the bottom, while the inferior wall is at the top. (LA: left atrium, LV: left ventricle, ALPM: anterolateral papillary muscle)

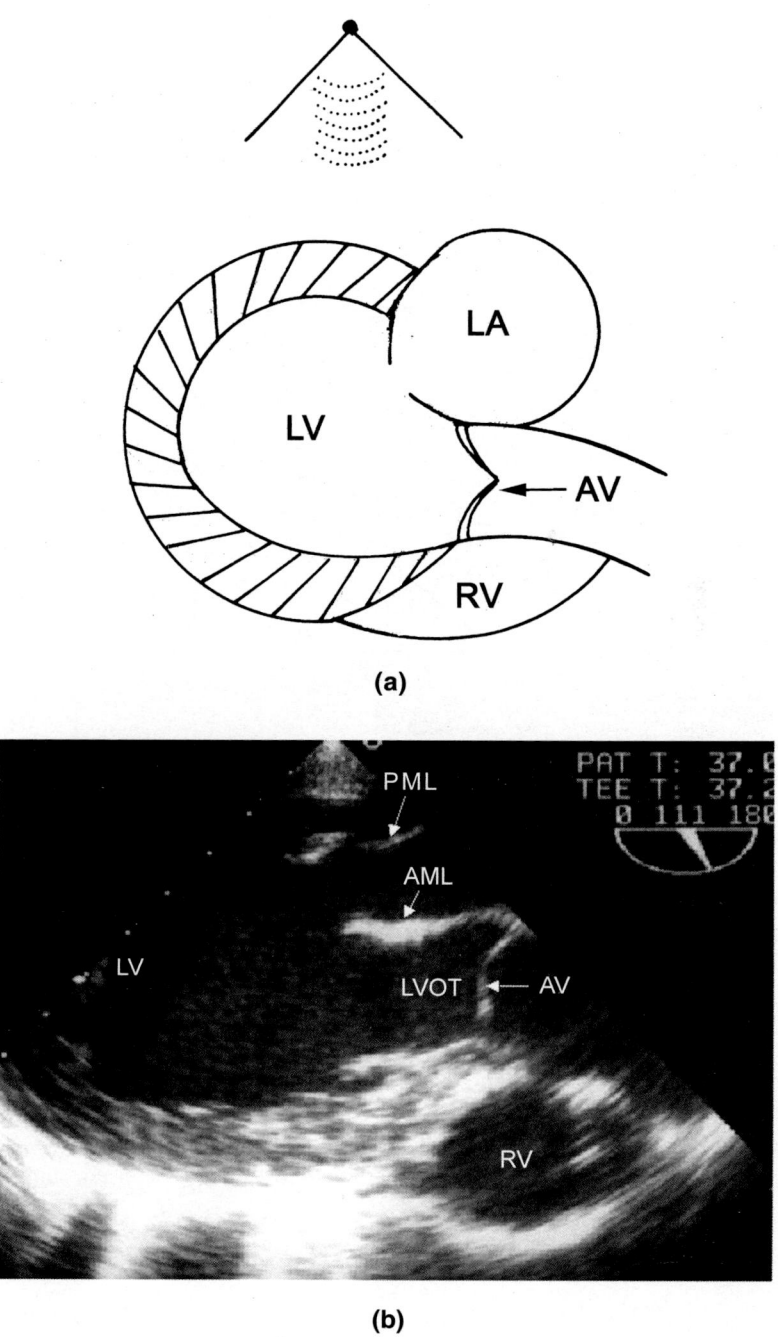

(a)

(b)

Figure 2.18 (a) Diagrammatic representation of longitudinal proximal transgastric view. **(b)** At 110 to 120 degrees the left ventricular outflow tract is seen to open into the aorta in its longitudinal course. This view can be used to evaluate the subvalvular apparatus of the mitral valve and the anterior and inferior wall of the left ventricle. (LA: left atrium, LV: left ventricle, AML: anterior mitral leaflet, PML: posterior mitral leaflet, LVOT: left ventricular outflow tract, AV: aortic valve, RV: right ventricle)

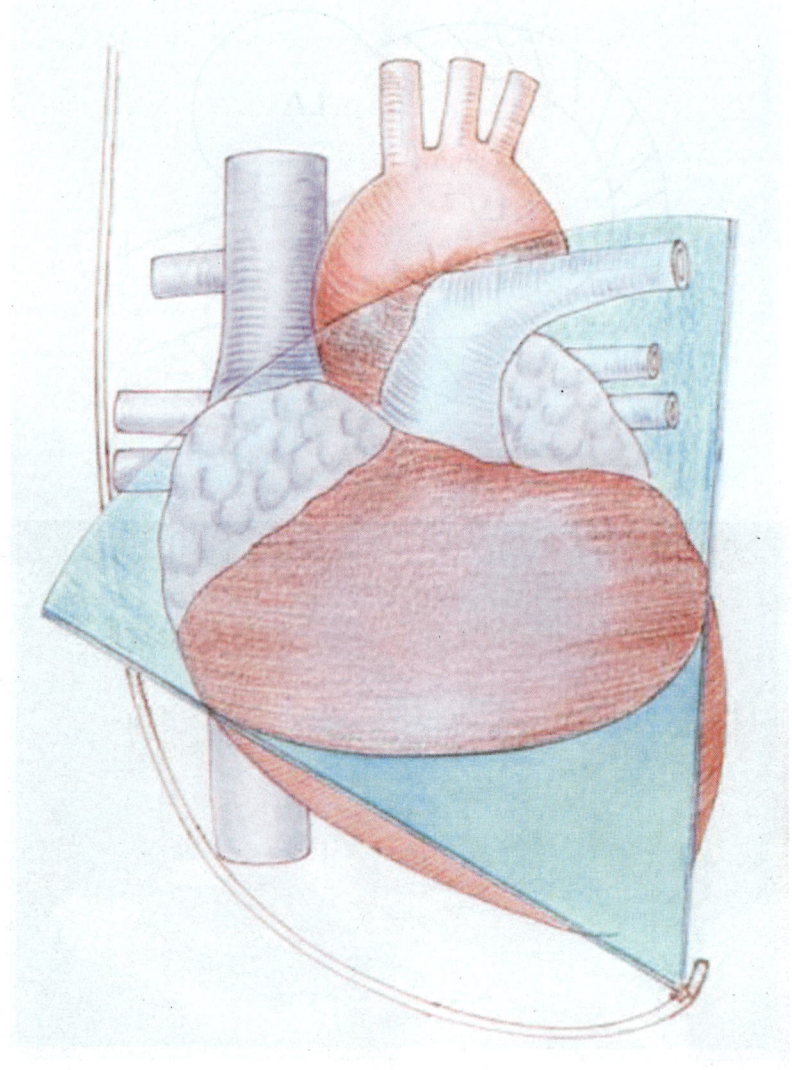

(a)

Figure 2.19. Deep transgastric view of the left ventricle.
(a) Diagrammatic representation of ultrasound beam.

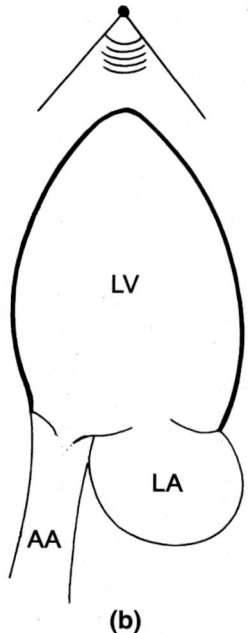

(b)

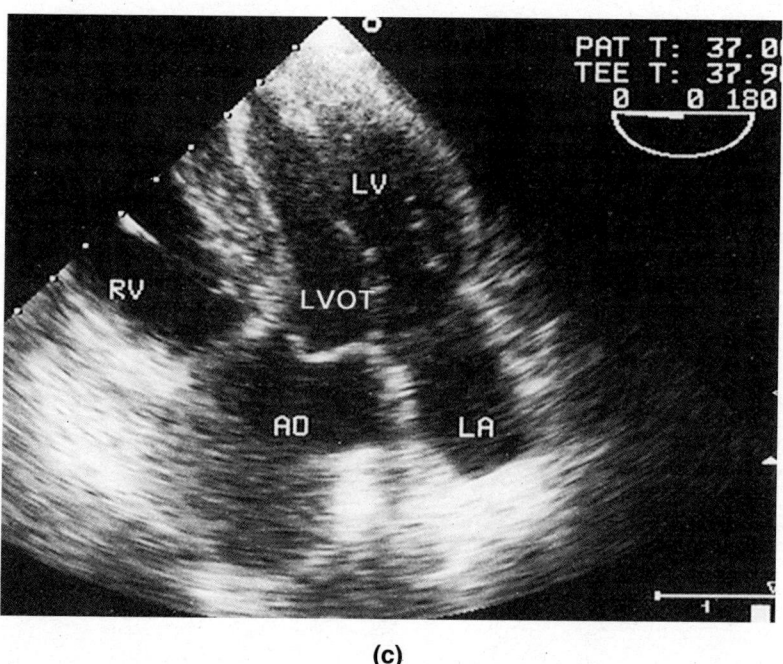

(c)

Figure 2.19 (b) Diagrammatic representation of ultrasound image. **(c)** With the imaging plane at 0°, a three chamber view with the left ventricular outflow tract, aortic valve and a proximal portion of ascending aorta in the centre (left of the left atrium) is obtained. As this view allows an excellent alignment of the ultrasound beam and the blood flow out of the left ventricle, it remains the best view for Doppler measurement of cardiac output and the Doppler quantification of aortic stenosis. (LV: left ventricle, LVOT: left ventricular outflow tract, AO: aorta, LA: left atrium, RV: right ventricle)

Chapter 3

EVALUATION OF THE LEFT VENTRICULAR FUNCTION

Evaluation of the left ventricular function

Transoesophageal echocardiography (TOE) has been used extensively for the evaluation of haemodynamic and global ventricular function. Standard haemodynamic variables, e.g. filling pressures and cardiac output, that are normally obtained by other invasive techniques such as pulmonary artery catheterisation, have been estimated with TOE. In addition, it has also been used to quantify cardiac dimension, intracardiac flow rates and overall cardiac performance.

Haemodynamic and other physiologic stresses during the perioperative period increase the risk of perioperative myocardial ischaemia. This is particularly true for patients with coronary artery disease or those who have multiple risk factors for coronary artery disease. The role of TOE for detecting ischaemia during both cardiac and noncardiac surgery is being increasingly recognised since traditional methods like ECG have a limited diagnostic accuracy. Detection of regional ventricular dysfunction can be useful for making therapeutic decisions like graft revisions and instituting haemodynamic supports in these patients. Such interventions improve the overall surgical success and outcome. Evaluation in multiple planes is required for delineating the area at risk. Interpretation of wall motion abnormalities however requires expertise. TOE provides a more accurate estimate of changes in preload and left ventricular filling pressures and thus is relatively easier and more accurate than pulmonary artery catheterisation. The diagnosis of haemodynamic problems such as hypovolaemia or myocardial dysfunction as a cause of decreased cardiac output, can be easily differentiated for choosing the right therapeutic options in the post operative period.

Anaesthesiologists with basic TOE training should be able to make a qualitative assessment of the haemodynamic status and myocardial function. TOE views providing information regarding cardiac geometry and dimensions are utilised for the estimation of preload, afterload and contractility. In addition, the estimation of diastolic function is performed by determining the pattern of left ventricular filling with the help of transmitral and pulmonary venous flow characteristics. In this chapter, the views used for calculation of the left ventricular dimensions and the Doppler flow patterns across the mitral valve and pulmonary veins are illustrated.

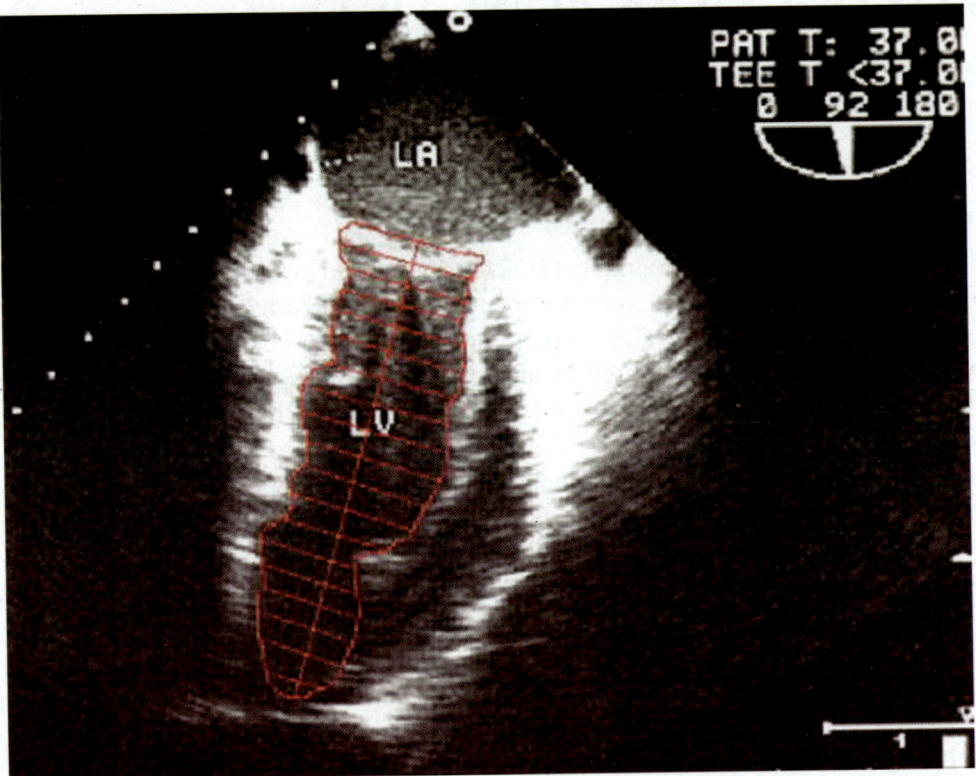

Figure 3.1. Two chamber view showing application of Simpson's rule to determine left ventricular volume off-line. According to this rule, planimetry (computer assisted) is used to outline the endocardial border in a longitudinal view. The software subsequently dissects the outlined area in a series of 20 ellipsoid cylinders of equal height. The sum of volumes of the individual slices gives the total chamber volume. (LA: left atrium, LV: left ventricle)

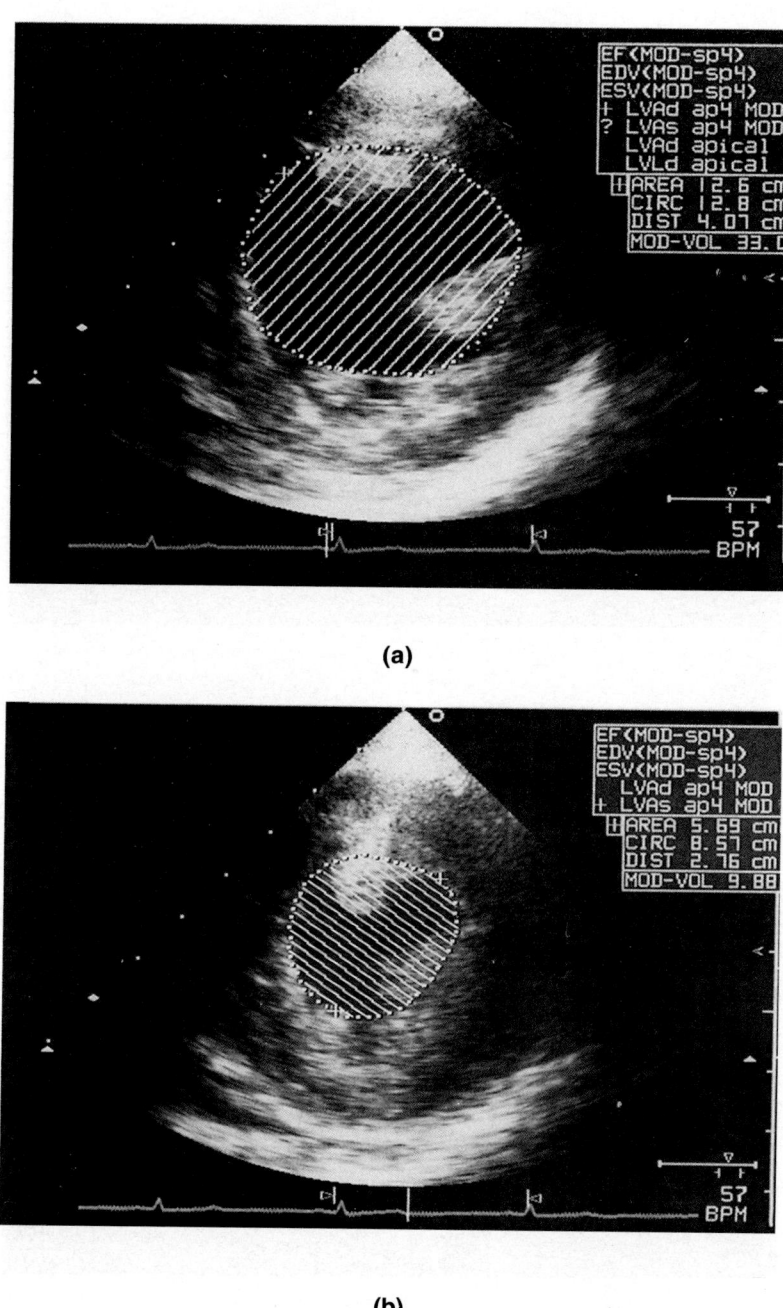

(a)

(b)

Figure 3.2 (a) Left ventricular end-diastolic area (LVEDA) is measured in the mid-papillary short axis view. Changes in the LVEDA consistently reflect the changes in the LV end-diastolic volume. Note that the papillary muscles are included in the LV endocardial outline. **(b)** shows the LV end-systolic area. The method helps to measure the ejection fraction.

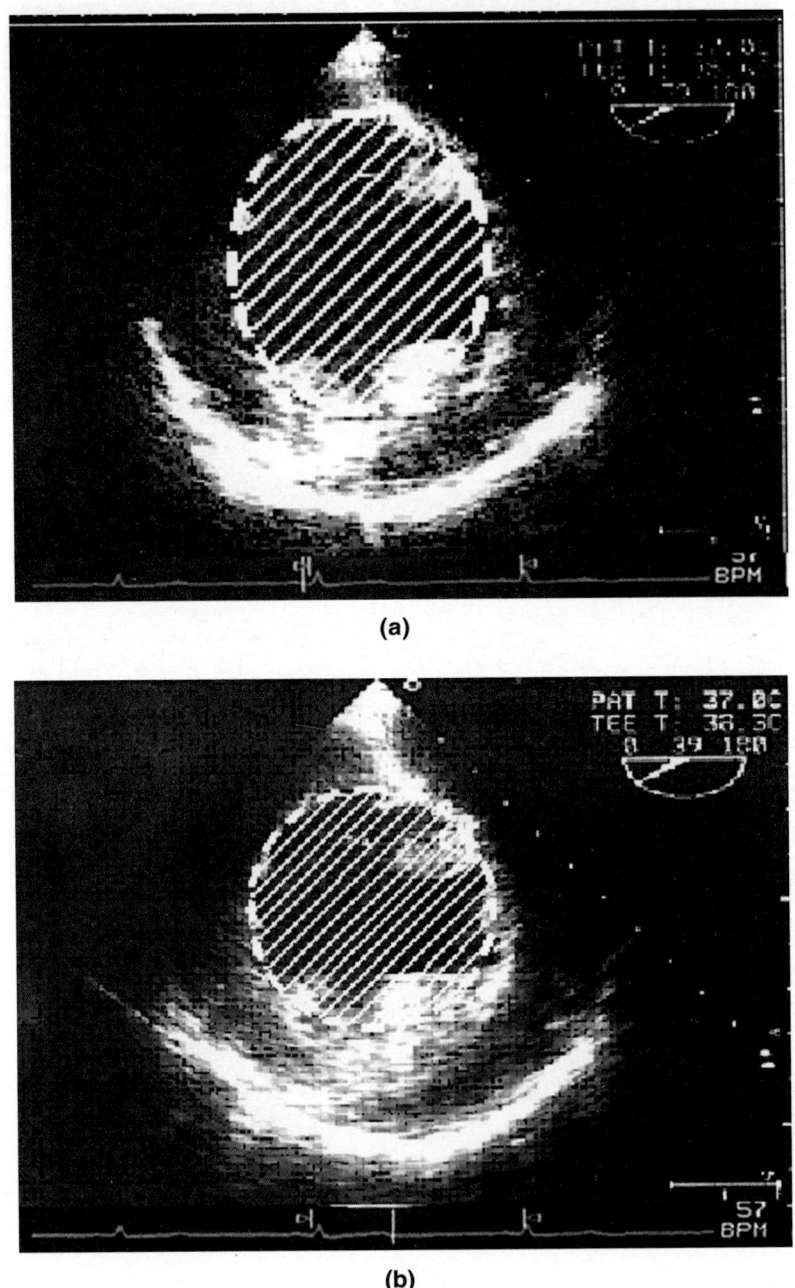

(a)

(b)

Figure 3.3. Mid-papillary short axis view of the left ventricle (LV) in a patient with LV dysfunction. Note the LV area in end-diastole **(a)** and end-systole **(b)**.

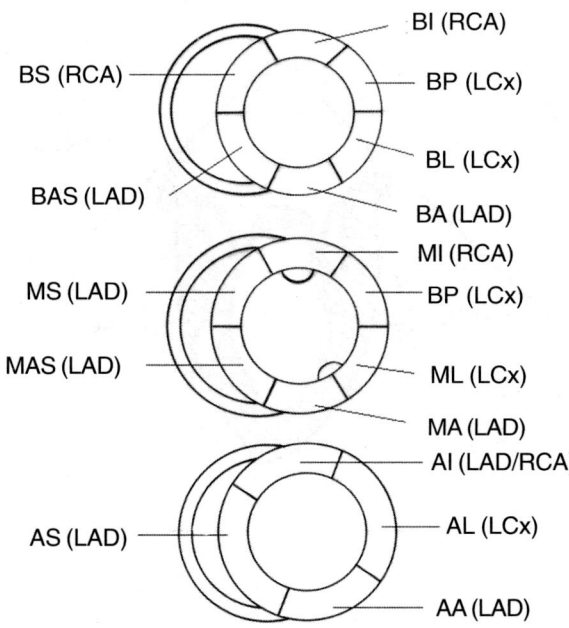

Figure 3.4. Diagrammatic representation of left ventricular segments. (BI: basal inferior, BP: basal posterior, BL: basal lateral, BA: basal anterior, BAS: basal anteroseptal, BS: basal septal, MI: mid inferior, MP: mid posterior, ML: mid lateral, MA: mid anterior, MAS: mid anteroseptal, MS: mid septal, AI: apical inferior, AL: apical lateral, AA: apical anterior, AS: apical septal, LAD: left anterior descending artery, LCx: left circumflex artery, RCA: right coronary artery)

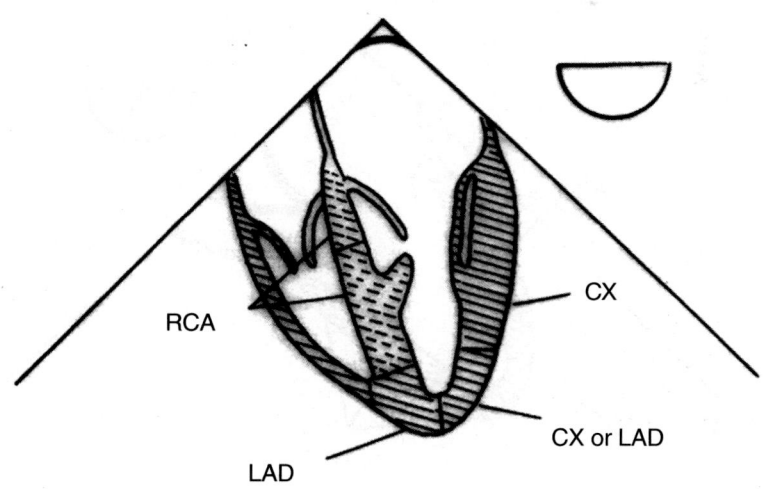

Figure 3.5. Diagrammatic representation of four chamber view illustrating the myocardial blood supply. (RCA: right coronary artery, LAD: left anterior descending coronary artery, CX: circumflex coronary artery)

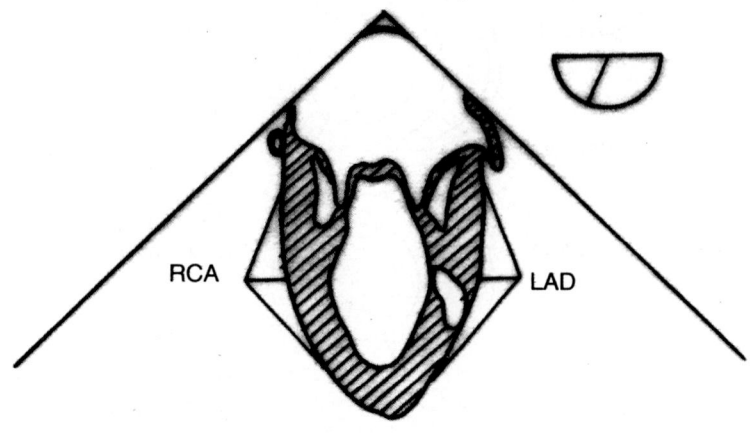

Figure 3.6. Diagrammatic representation of two chamber view illustrating the myocardial blood supply. (LAD: left anterior descending coronary artery, RCA: right coronary artery)

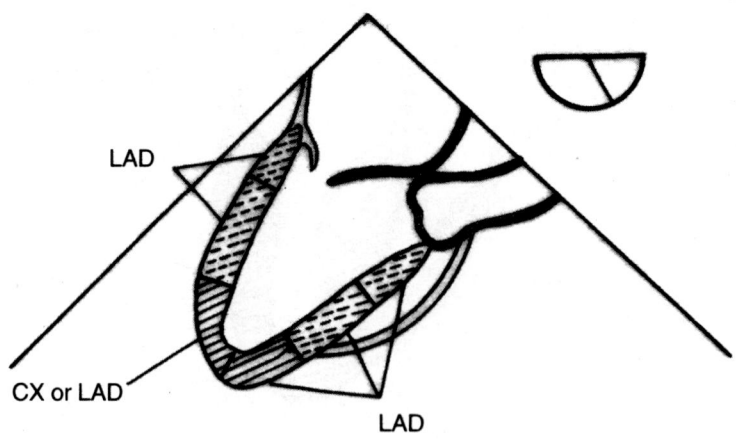

Figure 3.7. Diagrammatic representation of mid-axial long axis view illustrating myocardial blood supply. (LAD: left anterior descending coronary artery, CX: circumflex coronary artery)

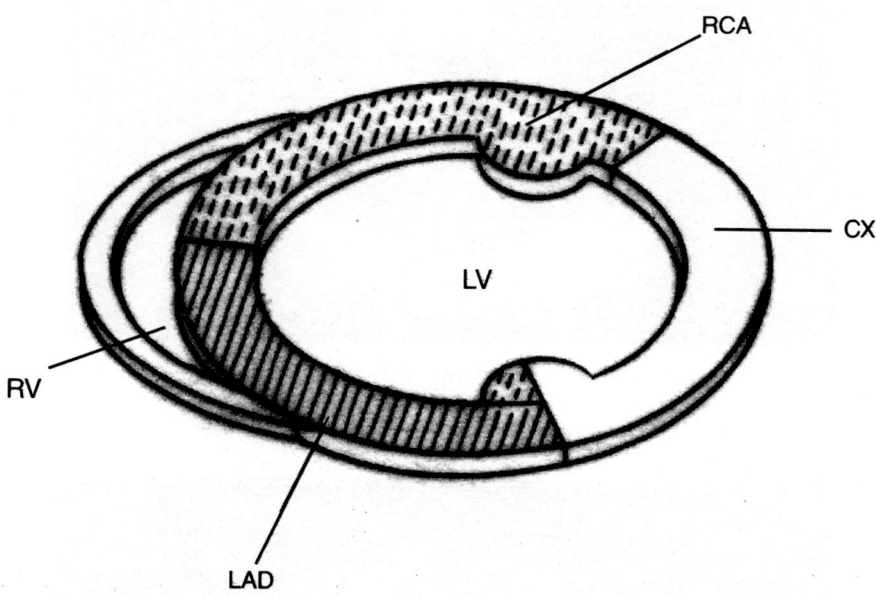

Figure 3.8. Diagrammatic representation of the short axis view of the left ventricle at midpapillary muscle level showing the coronary artery supply. (LAD: left anterior descending coronary artery, RCA: right coronary artery, CX: circumflex coronary artery, LV : left ventricle, RV : right ventricle)

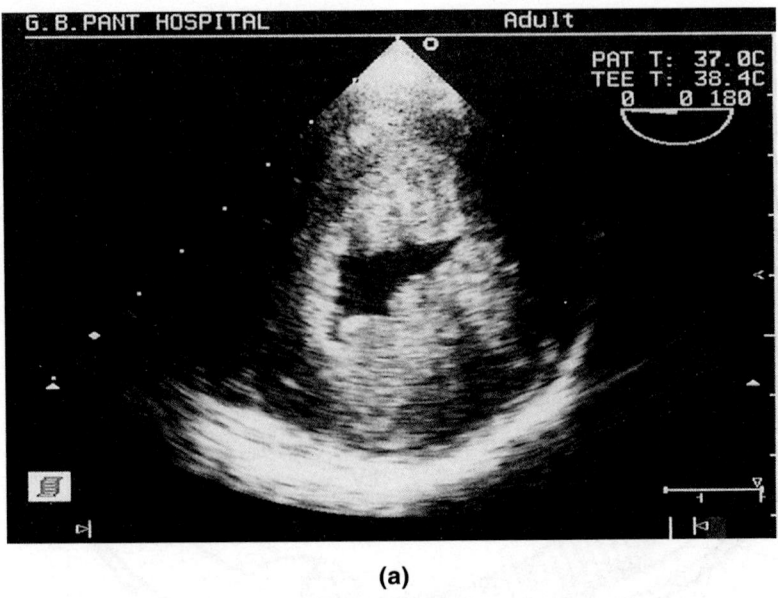

(a)

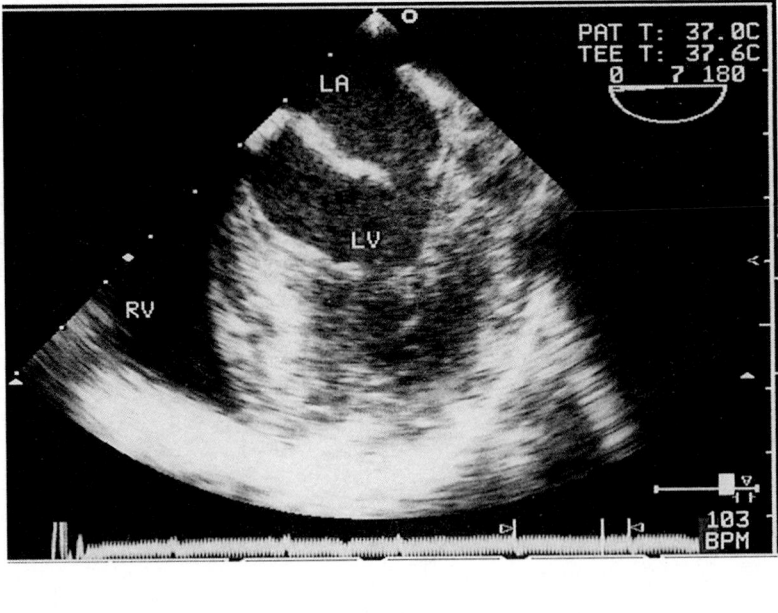

(b)

Figure 3.9. Left ventricular function assessment in a patient with aortic stenosis. Note the concentric left ventricular hypertrophy in transgastric short axis view **(a)** and four chamber view **(b)**. (LA: left atrium, LV: left ventricle, RV: right ventricle)

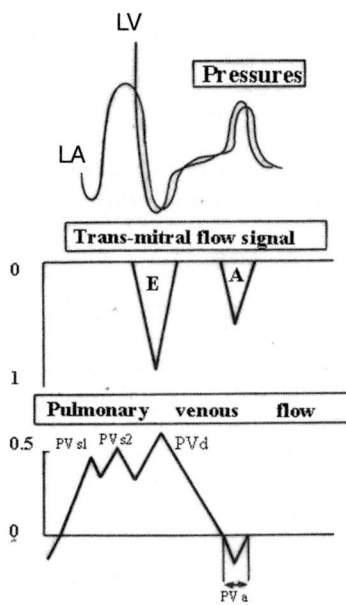

Figure 3.10. Assessment of diastolic function and left ventricular (LV) filling pressures can be made by simultaneously measuring the pattern of transmitral or pulmonary venous flow. This diagrammatic representation compares serial changes in transmitral flow and pulmonary vein Doppler flow with left atrial (LA) and LV pressures. (PVs1: peak flow velocity in early ventricular systole, PVs2: peak flow velocity later in systole, PVd: peak diastolic flow velocity, PVa: peak reverse flow velocity at atrial contraction, E: represents early rapid LV filling, A: late LV filling that corresponds to atrial contraction)

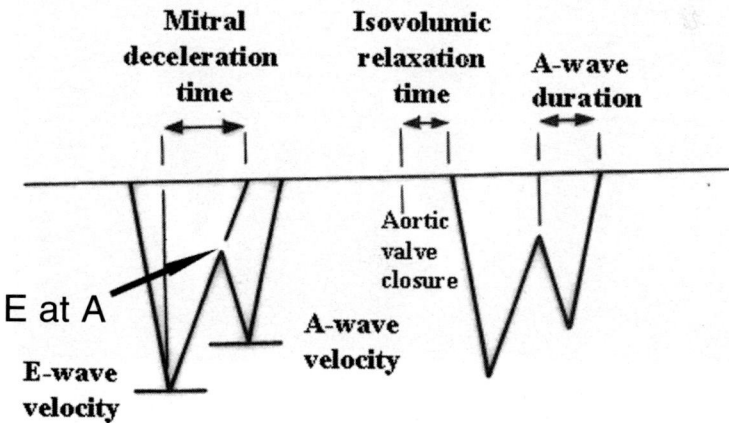

Figure 3.11. Clinical variables in transmitral flow. E represents the wave caused by transmitral flow in early diastole while A represents flow caused by atrial contraction. E at A is the mitral flow velocity at the onset of atrial contraction.

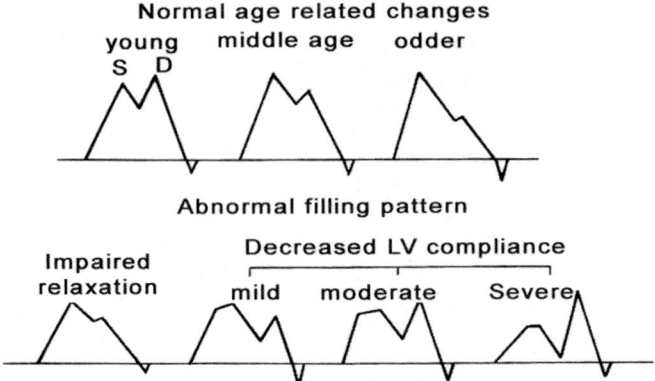

Figure 3.12. Diagrammatic representation of normal and abnormal pulmonary venous flow signals. At young age, the systolic (S) and diastolic (D) flow velocites are nearly equal. As the age advances, the systolic velocity increases and the diastolic velocity decreases.

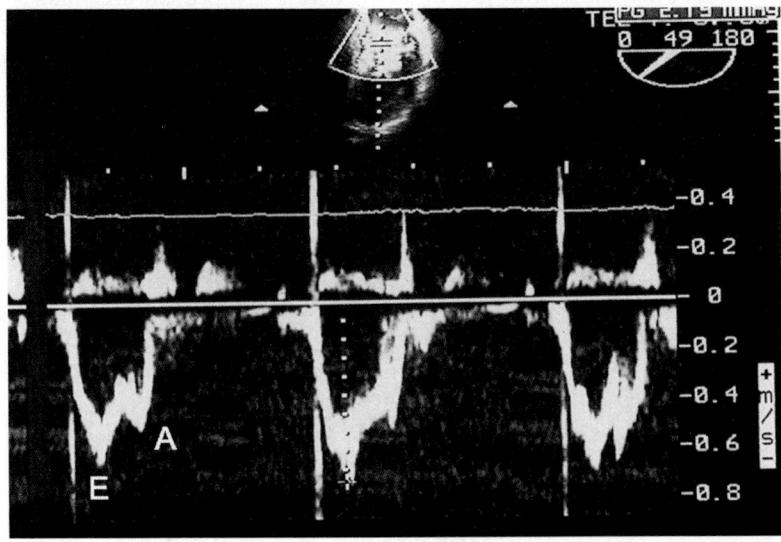

Figure 3.13. Trans-mitral flow on pulsed wave Doppler in a patient with normal left ventricular function. Note the early diastolic filling (E) and late diastolic filling (A) waves, with a normal E/A ratio (>1)

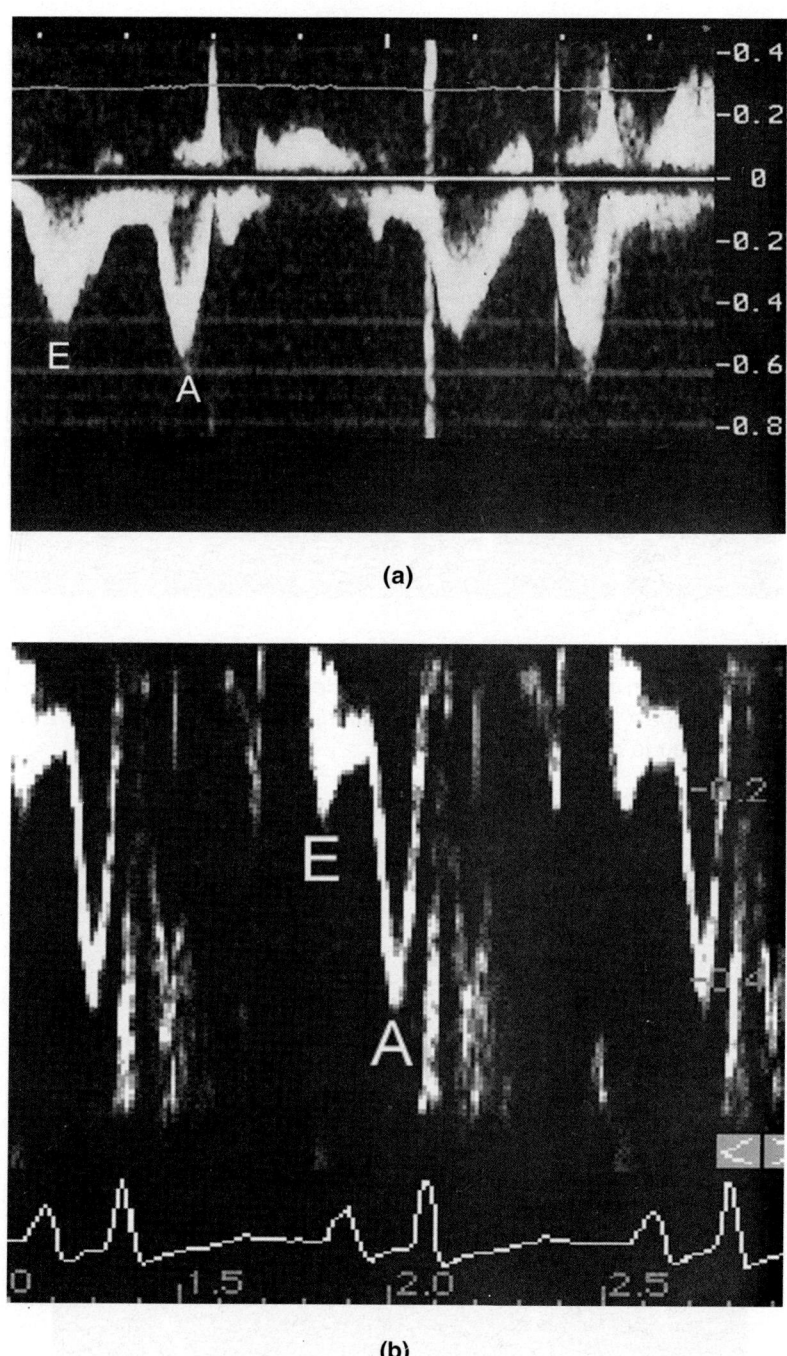

Figure 3.14 (a & b) Mitral inflow pulsed wave Doppler in two patients with diastolic dysfunction (grade I). Note the taller late diastolic filling wave (A) caused by the exaggerated atrial contraction (E/A ratio <1)

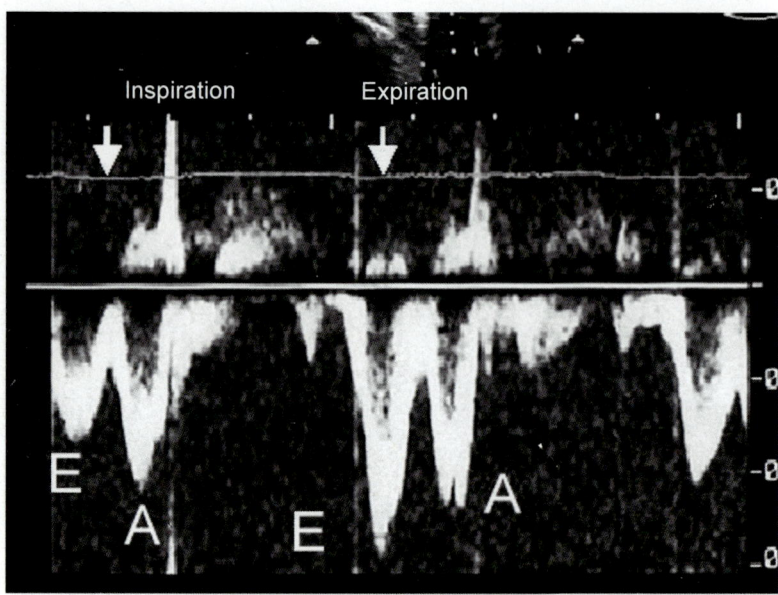

Figure 3.15. Trans-mitral pulsed wave Doppler flow pattern in a patient with diastolic dysfunction. E/A ratio in the first beat shows grade I dysfunction (E/A<1). With increase in the left atrial preload, at the onset of expiration, there is a change to a more normal looking pattern (pseudo-normal, grade II).

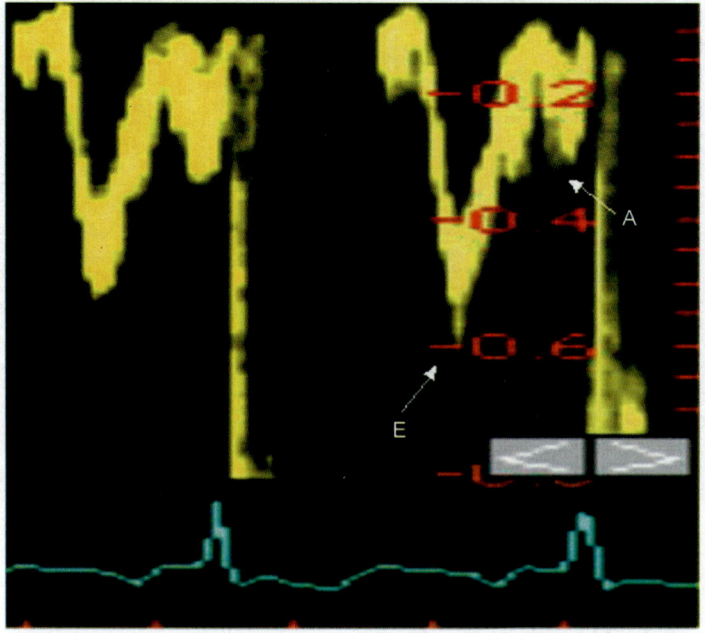

Figure 3.16. Transmitral flow pattern in a patient with severe diastolic dysfunction. Note the E/A>2 (Grade III) with a E wave deceleration time of 100 ms.

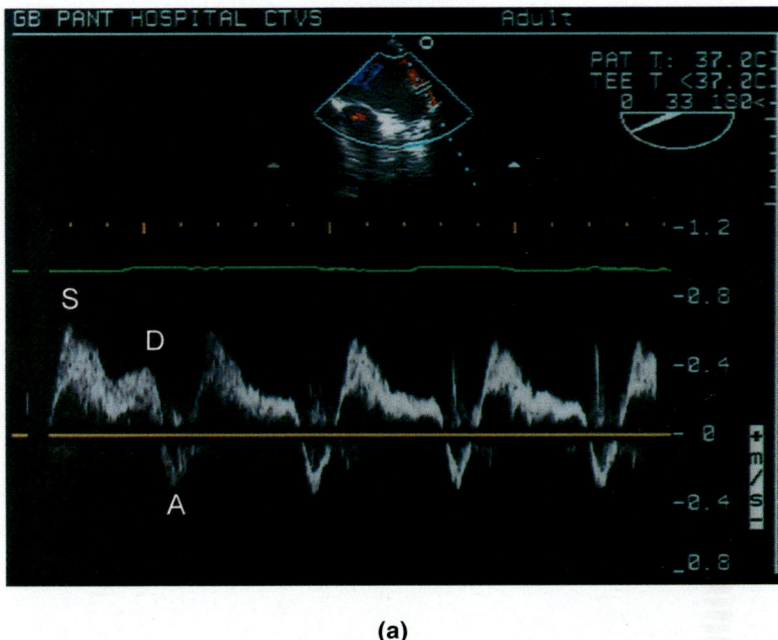

(a)

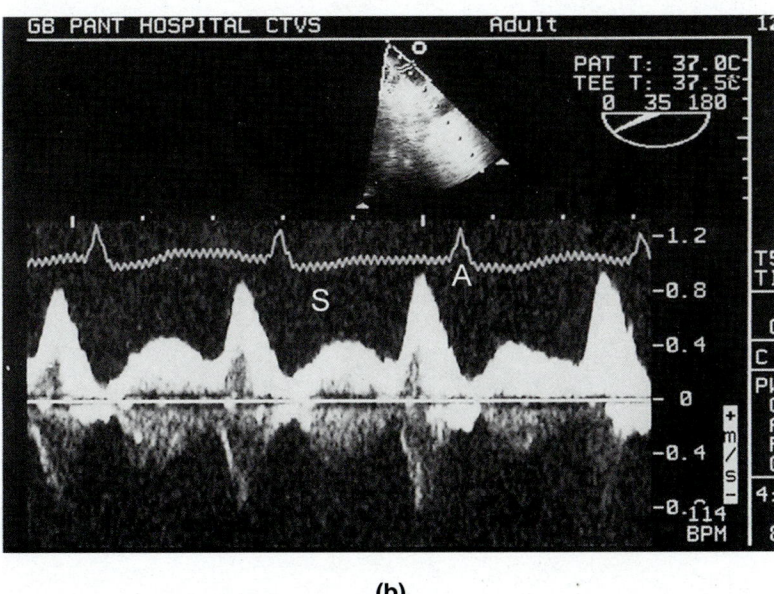

(b)

Figure 3.17 (a) Pulsed wave Doppler from pulmonary vein for estimating left ventricular filling pressures. Note the normal waveforms (antegrade systolic- S, diastolic- D and retrograde A wave). **(b)** Shows waveforms in a patient with severe diastolic dysfunction. Note the attenuated forward flow in early and mid-diastole and exaggerated flow in late diastole leading to reversed pattern of A wave.

Chapter 4

EVALUATION OF THE MITRAL VALVE

The potential for suboptimal surgical outcome is always present in patients undergoing valvular surgery. It is important to recognise the need for additional corrections in the immediate post-operative period. Transoesophageal echocardiography (TOE) during valvular surgery is, therefore, widely used in this setting.

TOE constitutes an important tool for assessing the mitral valve and provides an excellent anatomical visualisation, clear delineation of transmitral flow, and is highly sensitive for detecting valve regurgitation. It plays an important role in the accurate assessment of the mitral valve function, especially following valve replacement and repair. In addition, it reliably detects left atrial thrombi and vegetations. Before initiating cardiopulmonary bypass (CPB), TOE at times can detect thrombi and vegetations and this is important for modifying surgical strategies. In post CPB period, TOE can identify significant valve dysfunction (if present) for necessitating additional surgical correction. It should be remembered however, that post-CPB, detection of valvular regurgitation is confounded by mitral leakage that occurs in the presence of abnormal loading conditions or due to myocardial ischaemia. This needs to be kept in consideration before additional therapeutic strategies are initiated.

In this chapter, the illustrations demonstrate the various abnormalities of the mitral valve (stenosis and regurgitation). In addition, the colour Doppler images showing the flow patterns in these conditions have been shown. TOE can also be used during percutaneous transluminal mitral commissurotomy, which is a commonly performed procedure for patients with mitral stenosis. Images demonstrating the use of TOE during mitral commissurotomy have also been included.

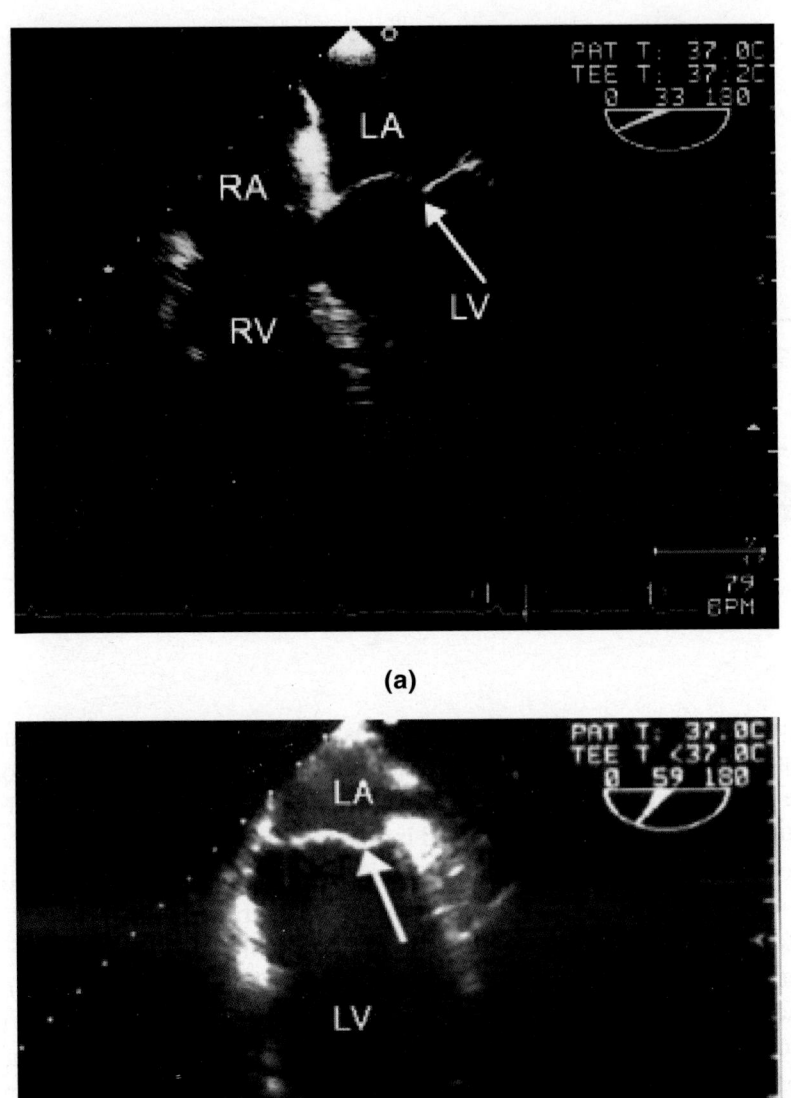

Figure 4.1. Appearance of the mitral valve on two-dimensional echo in four **(a)** and two **(b)** chamber views. Note the proper coaptation of the leaflets (arrow) during diastole. (LA: left atrium, RA: right atrium, LV: left ventricle, RV: right ventricle)

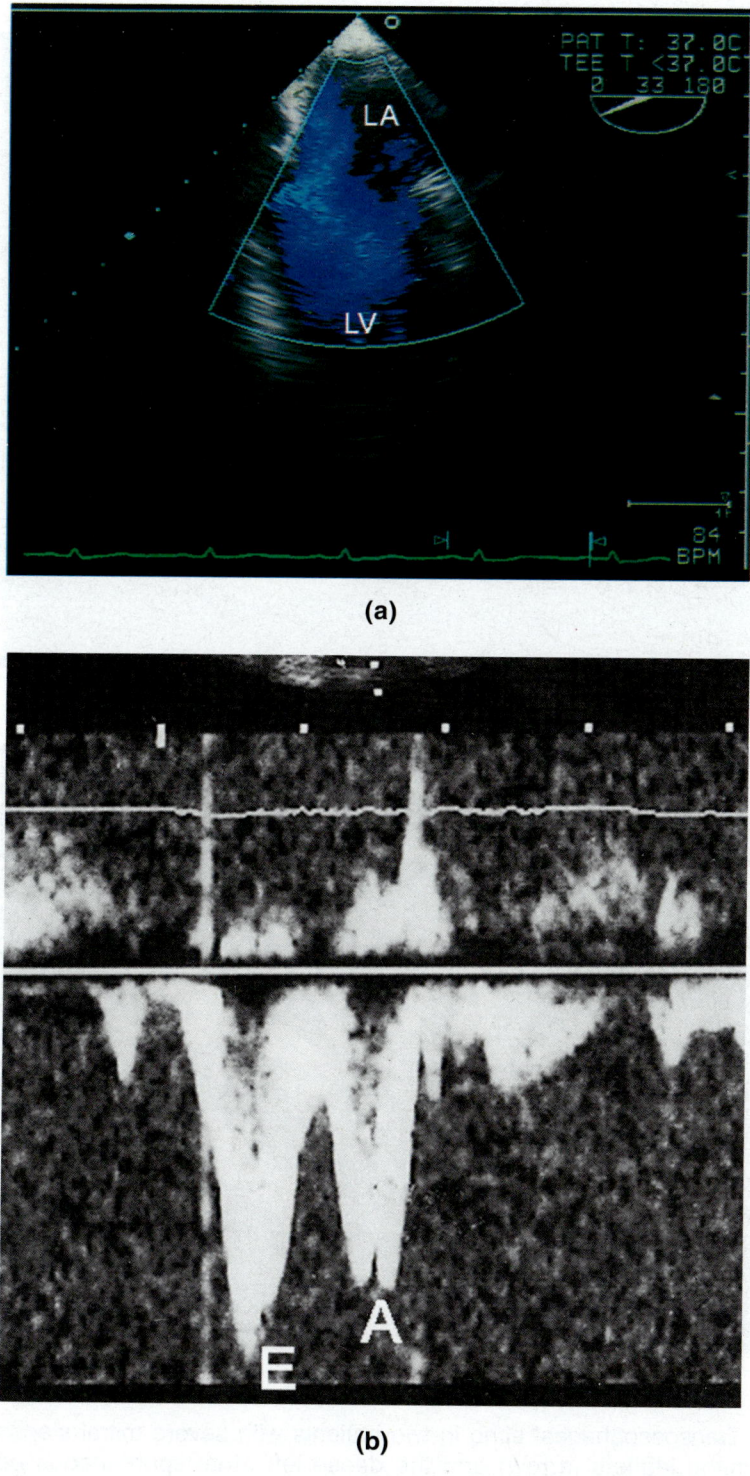

Figure 4.2. Normal trans-mitral flow on colour Doppler imaging **(a)** and pulsed Doppler imaging **(b)** (E- early diastolic flow, A- late diastolic flow, LA: left atrium, LV: left ventricle)

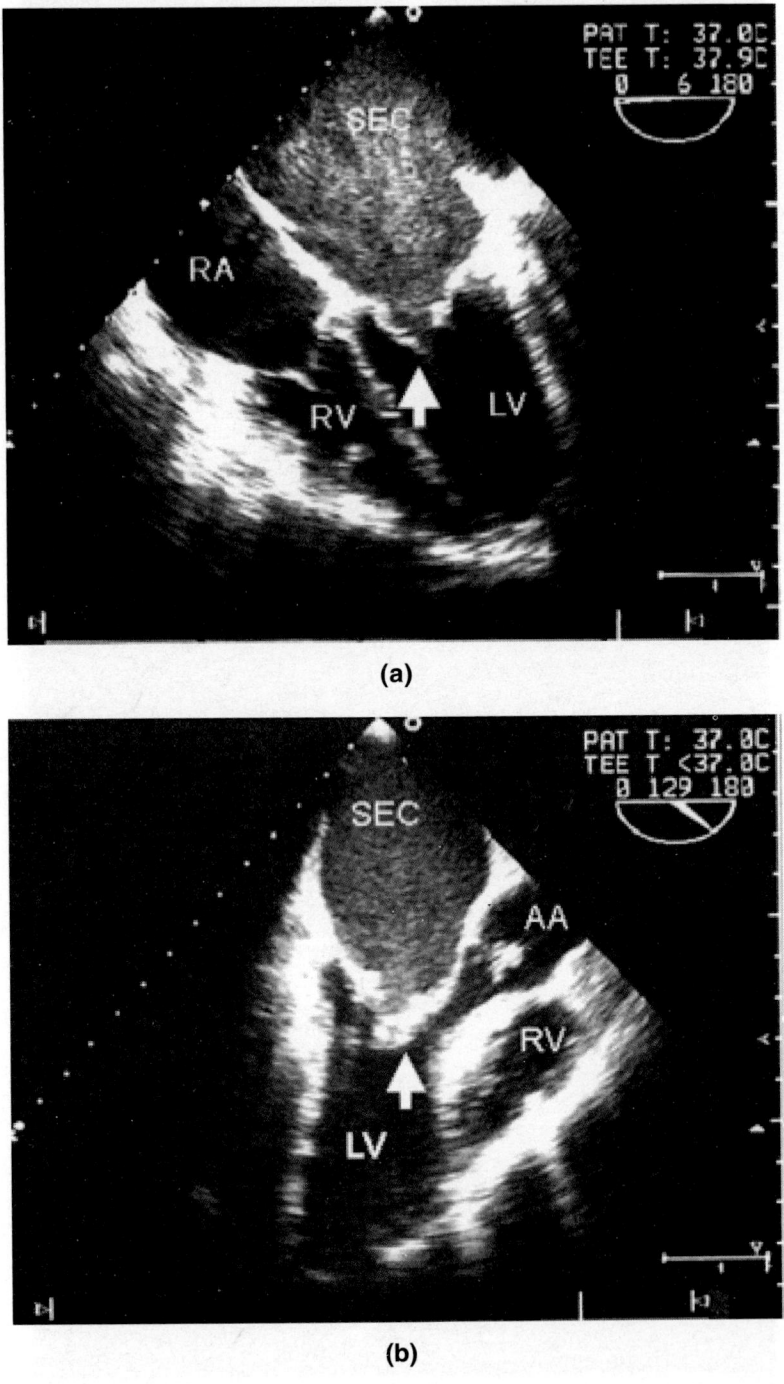

(a)

(b)

Figure 4.3. Transoesophageal echo in two patients with severe mitral stenosis. Note the doming of mitral leaflets (arrow) and the dense left atrial spontaneous echo contrast (SEC) in **(a & b)**. (RA: right atrium, RV: right ventricle, LV: left ventricle, AA: ascending aorta)

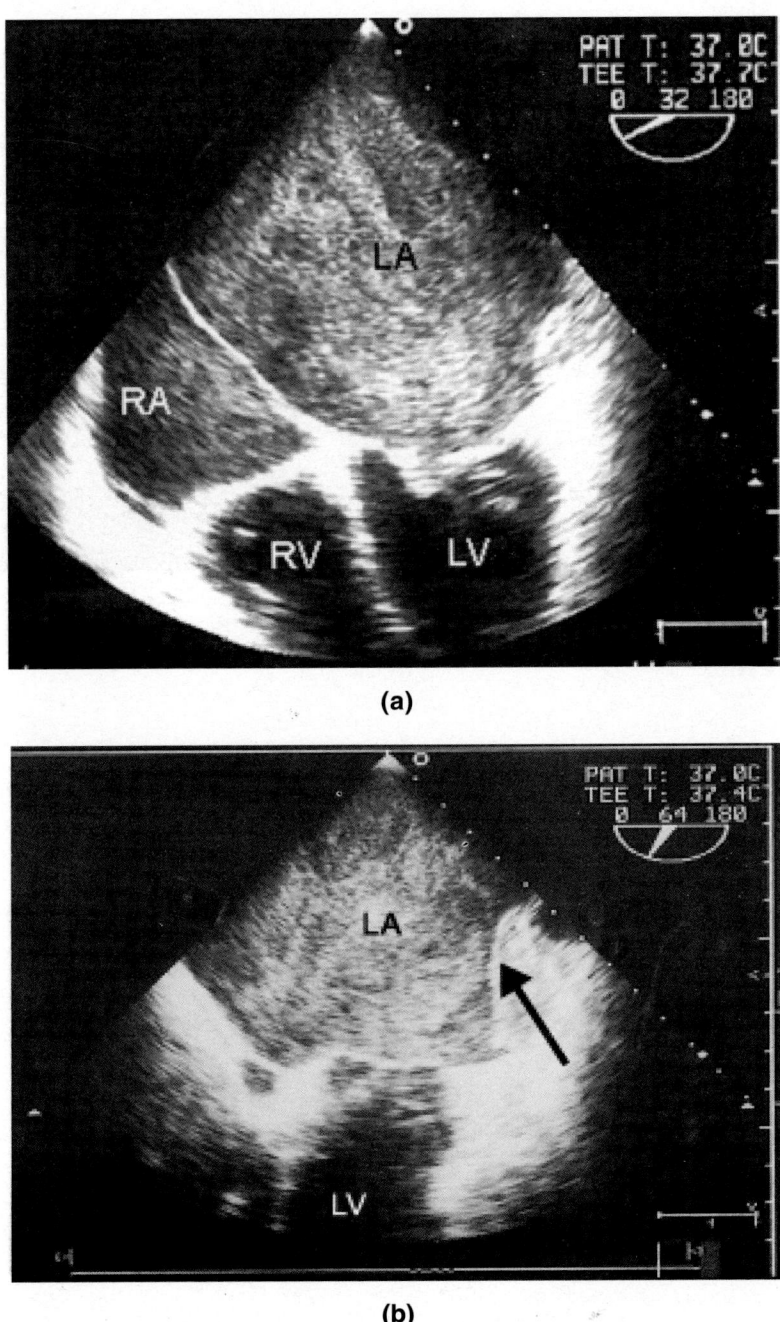

Figure 4.4. The appearance of left atrium in four chamber view **(a)** and two chamber view **(b)** in a patient with mitral stenosis. Note the bulging inter-atrial septum and the dense spontaneous left atrial contrast in the four chamber view and a well formed left atrial body clot (arrow) in the two chamber view. (LA : left atrium, RA : right atrium, RV : right ventricle, LV : left ventricle)

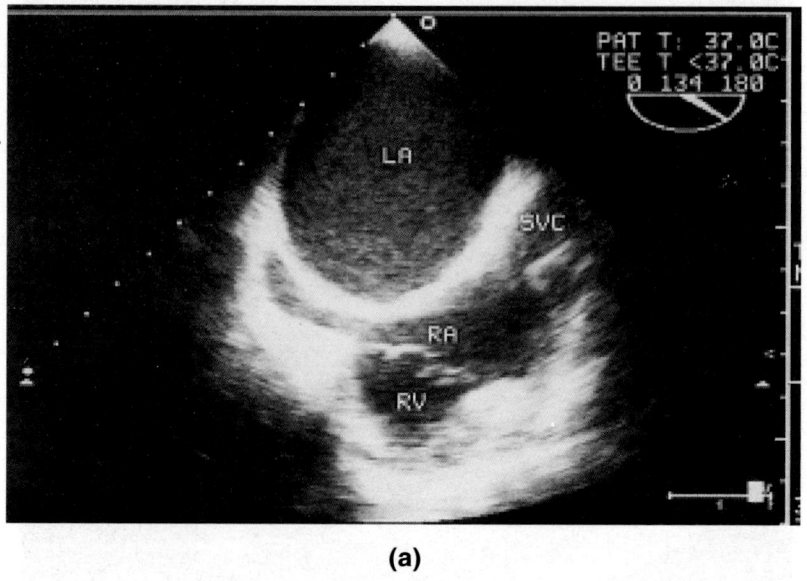

(a)

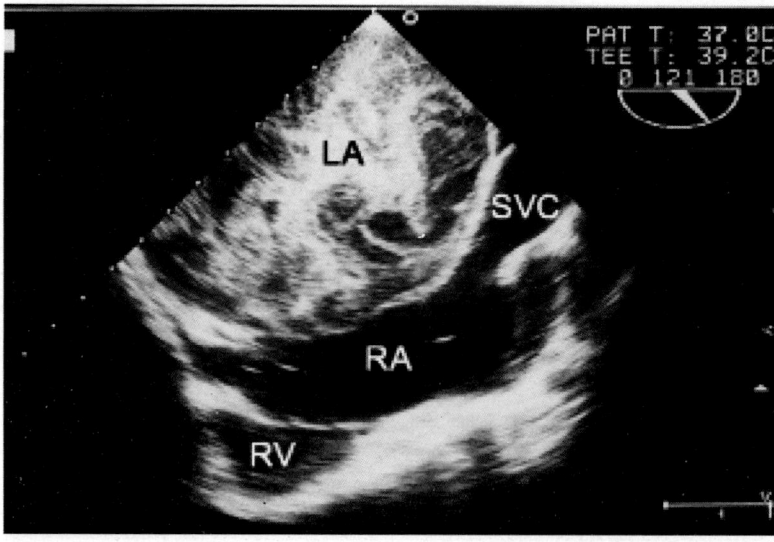

(b)

Figure 4.5 (a & b) Bicaval view of the left atrium in mitral stenosis. Note the difference in the size of the atrium in the two patients. Left atrium of the patient in (b) is larger and shows denser spontaneous echo contrast. (LA: left atrium, RA: right atrium, RV: right ventricle, SVC: superior vena cava)

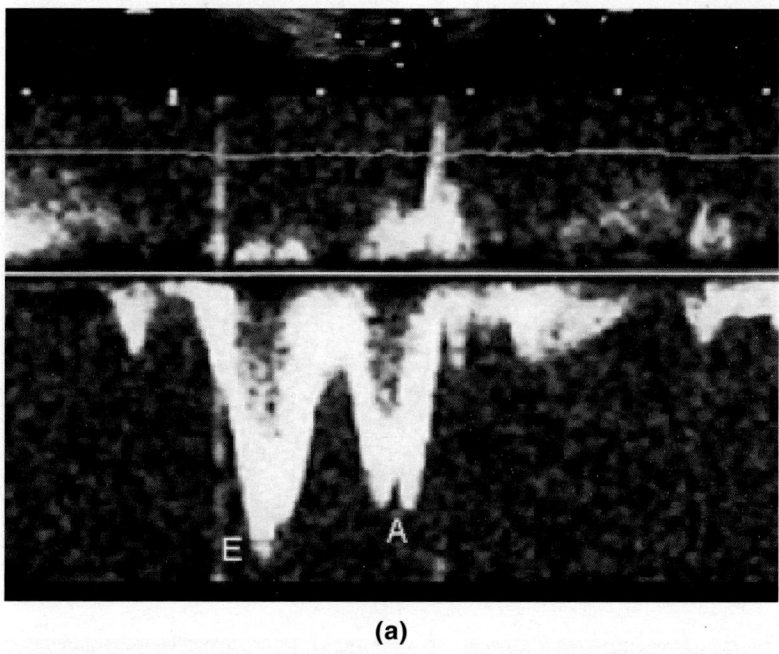

(a)

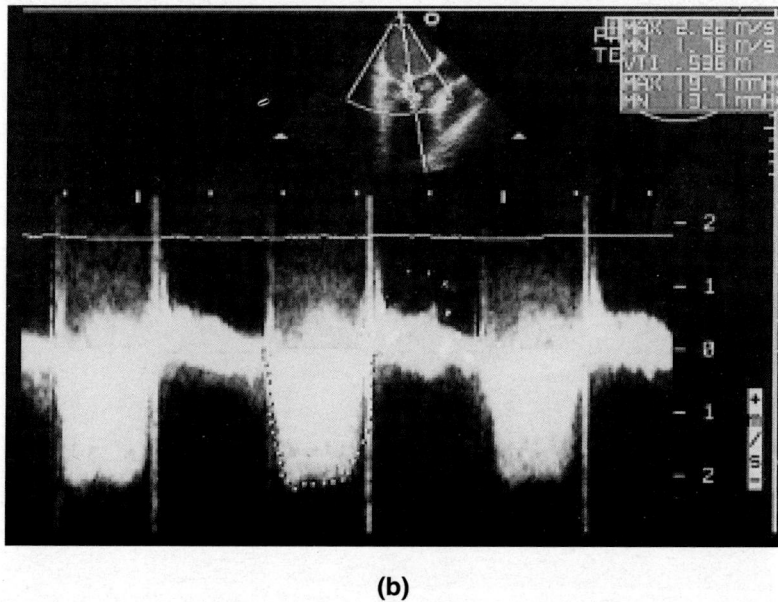

(b)

Figure 4.6. Pulsed wave Doppler across the mitral valve. **(a)** shows a bimodal flow in a normal person (E- early diastolic flow and A- late diastolic flow due to atrial contraction). **(b)** shows the continuous wave Doppler across the mitral valve in a patient with severe mitral stenosis. The spectral envelope in this view can be traced for calculating peak and mean mitral gradients.

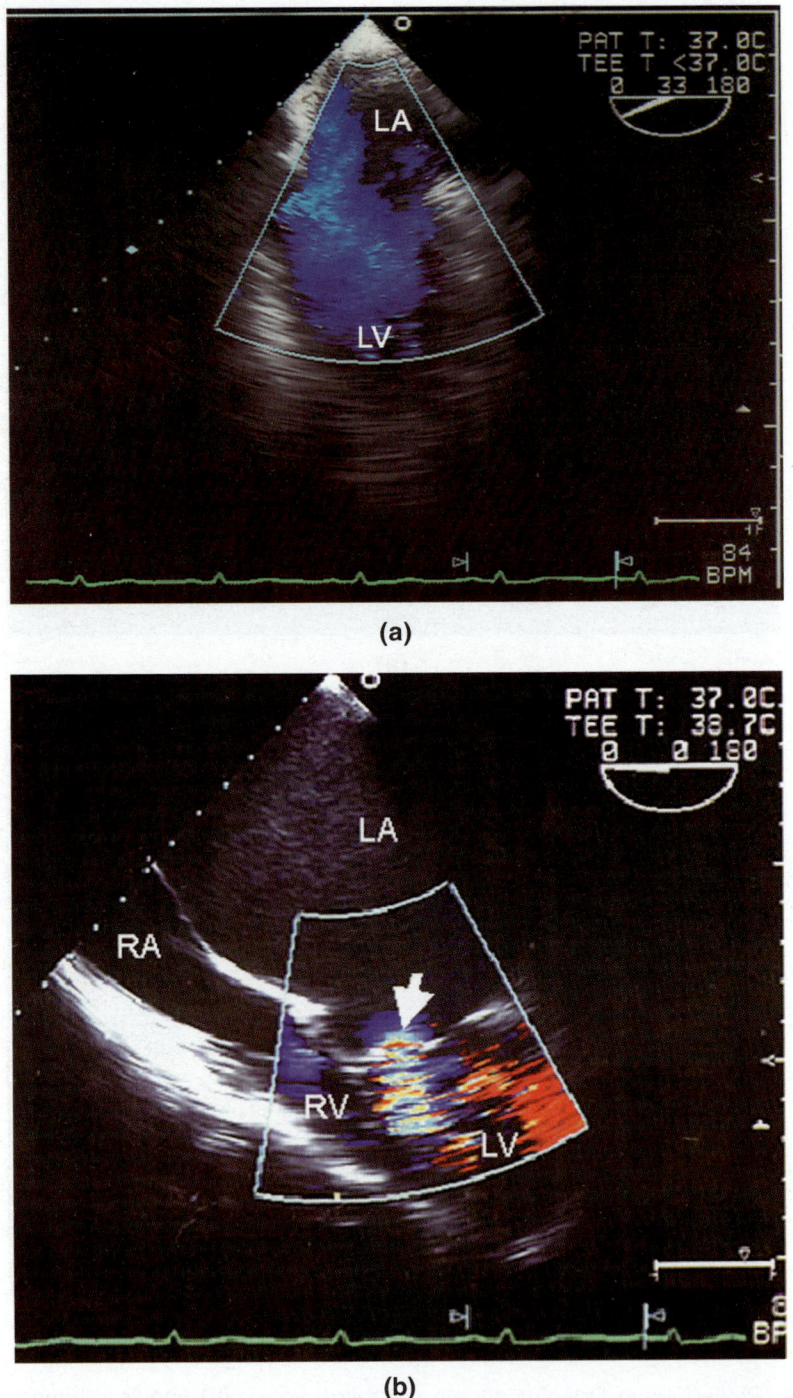

(a)

(b)

Figure 4.7 (a) Transmitral flow in a normal patient. Colour flow shows a low velocity, laminar non-turbulent flow. **(b)** shows the turbulent trans-mitral diastolic flow (arrow) in a patient with severe mitral stenosis. (LA: left atrium, LV: left ventricle, RA: right atrium, RV: right ventricle)

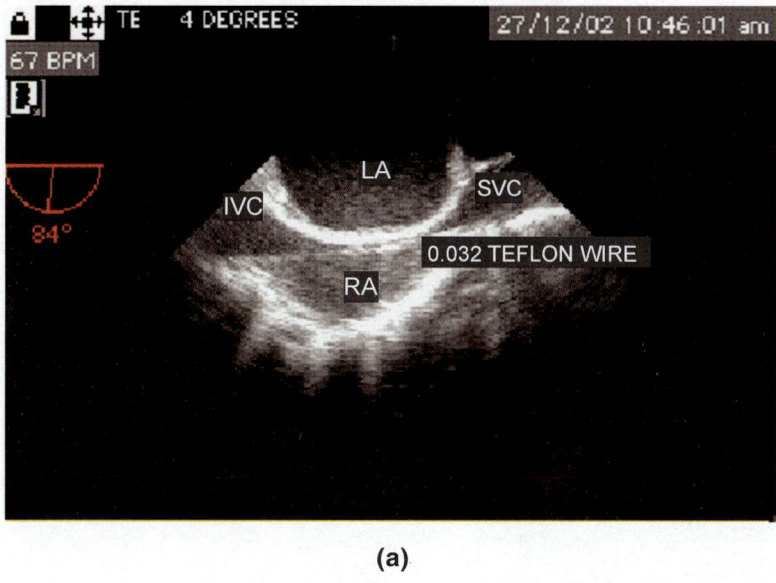

(a)

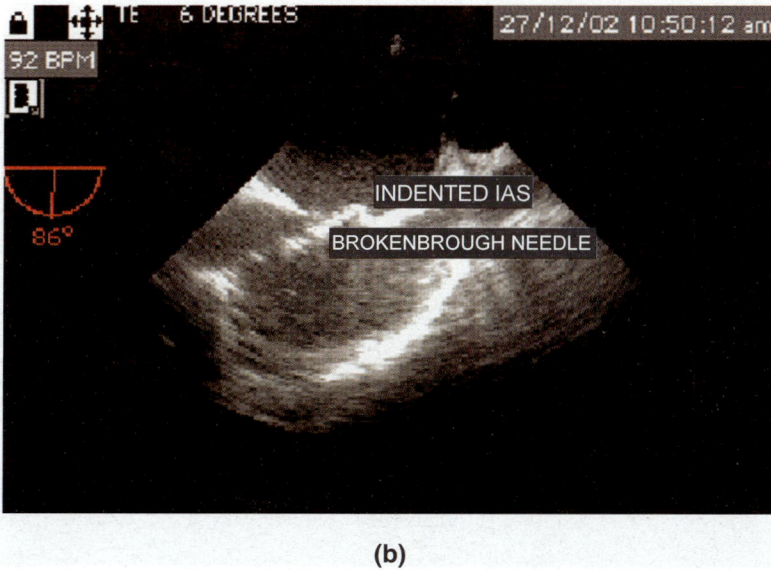

(b)

Figure 4.8. Use of transoesophageal echo for guiding percutaneous balloon mitral valvuloplasty.

(a) Bicaval view shows the placement of a 0.032 wire in the inferior vena cava used for placing Mullin's sheath. A trans-septal needle is introduced into this sheath and the entire assembly is moved down to a desirable point on the inter-atrial septum **(b)**. (LA: left atrium, RA : right atrium, SVC : superior vena cava, IVC : inferior vena cava)

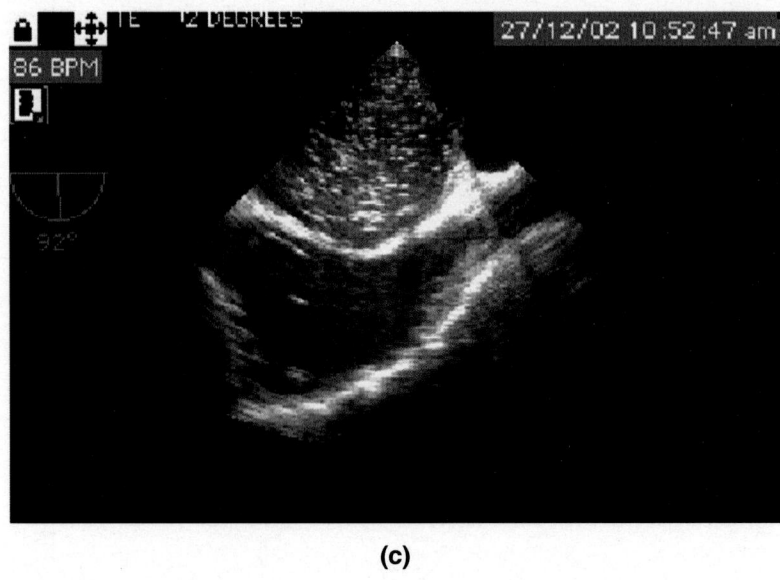

(c)

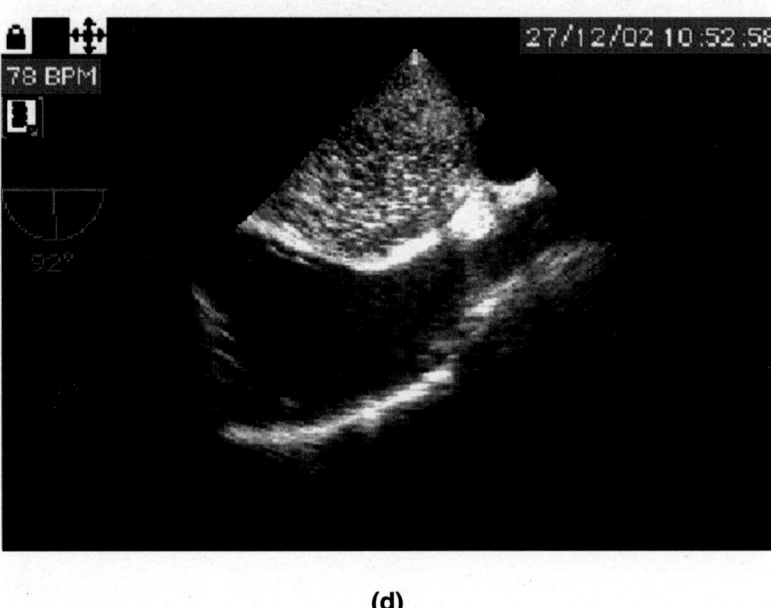

(d)

Figure 4.8 (c & d) Inter-atrial septum is punctured and the position of the needle inside the left atrium is confirmed by injecting saline contrast which opacifies the left atrium.

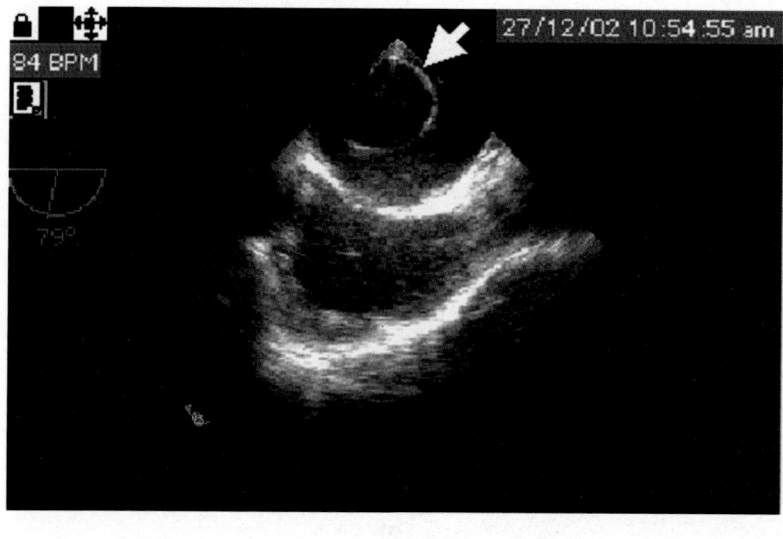

(e)

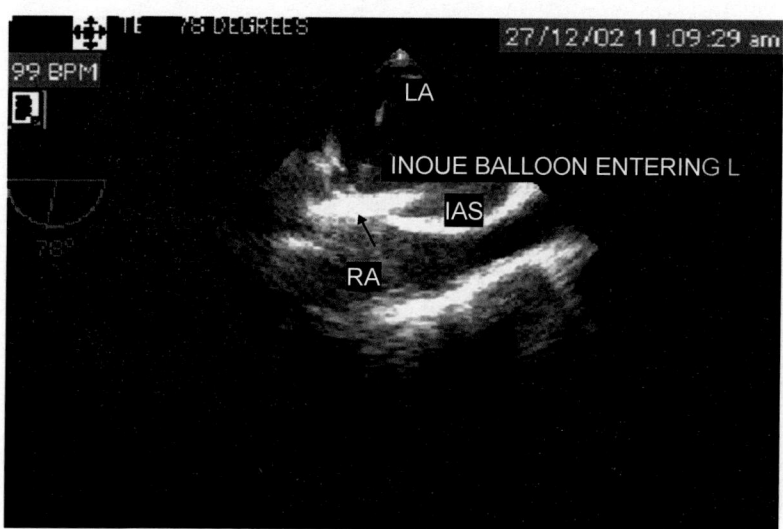

(f)

Figure 4.8. The trans-septal needle is removed, keeping the Mullin's sheath in place and a coil wire is introduced in the left atrium (arrow) **(e)**. The Mullin's sheath is removed keeping the coil wire in the left atrium, inter-atrial septum puncture site is dilated with a dilator and a Inoue balloon is introduced (arrow) **(f)** in its place over the coil wire.

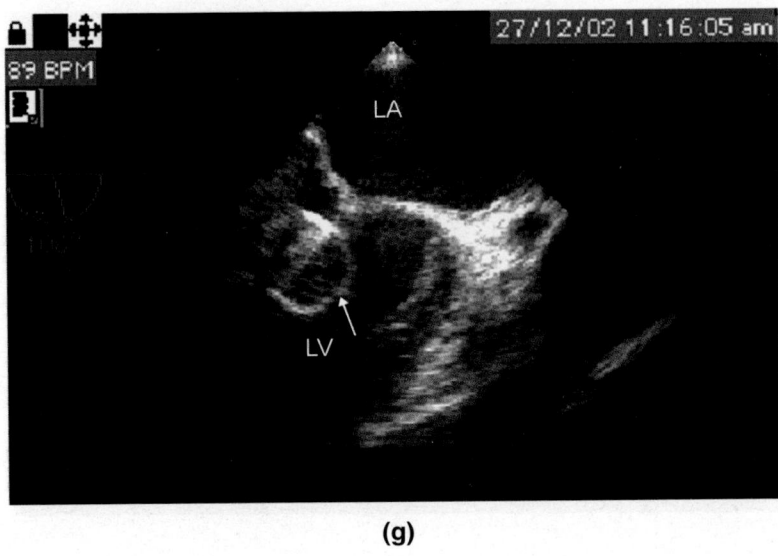

(g)

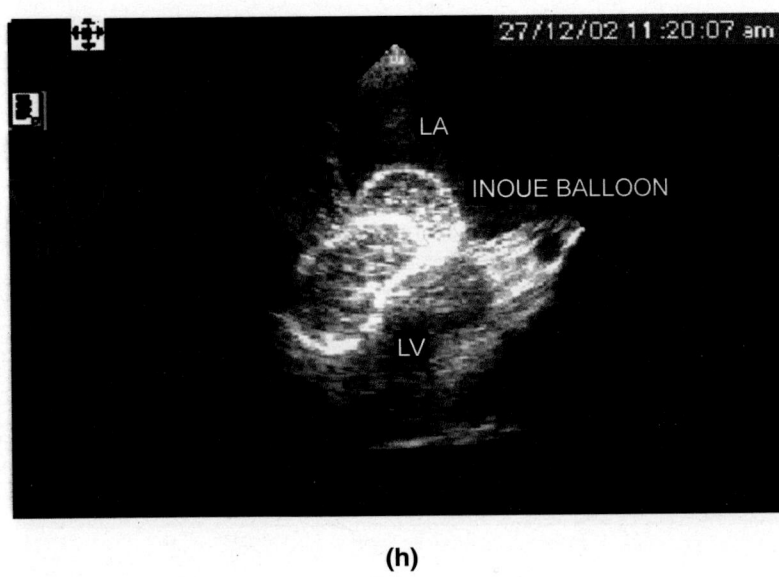

(h)

Figure 4.8 (g) The Inoue balloon is negotiated across the stenotic mitral valve (two chamber view). **(g)** The partly inflated balloon (arrow) is then pulled back across the mitral valve and **(h)** inflated completely for dilating the mitral valve. (LA: left atrium, LV: left ventricle)

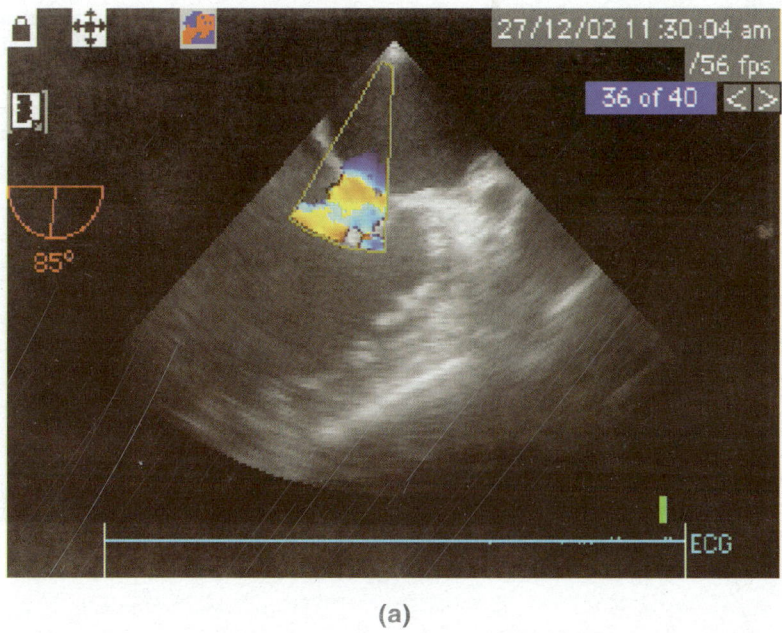

(a)

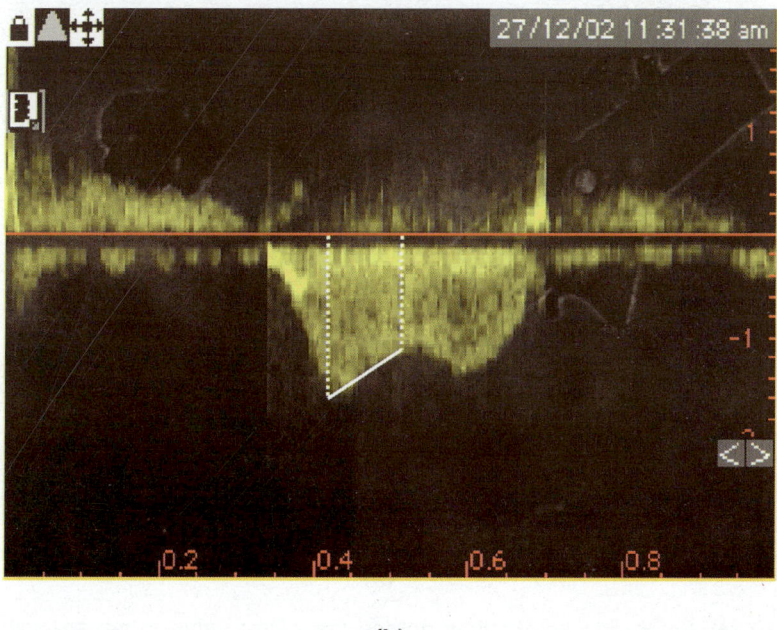

(b)

Figure 4.9 (a) Antegrade transmitral colour flow in a patient with severe mitral stenosis. **(b)** Continuous wave Doppler across the mitral valve is used for calculating severity of the mitral stenosis by knowing the deceleration slope (pressure half time-method).

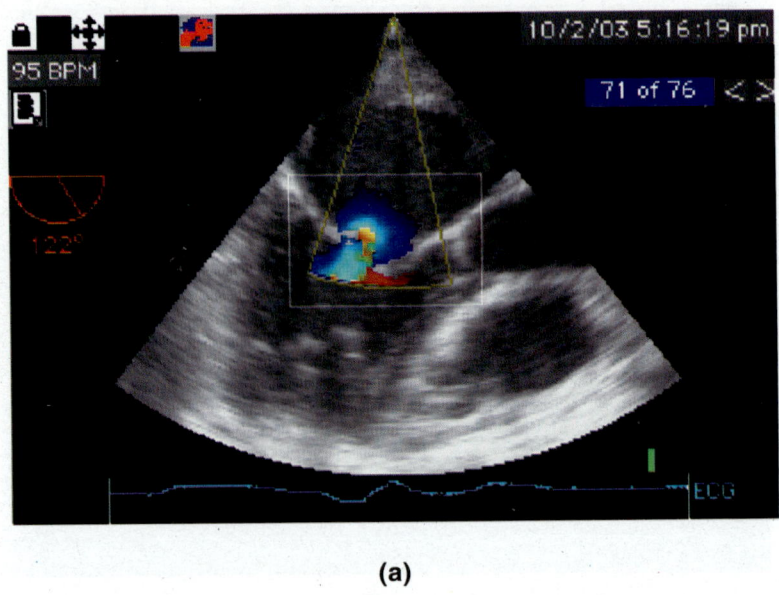

(a)

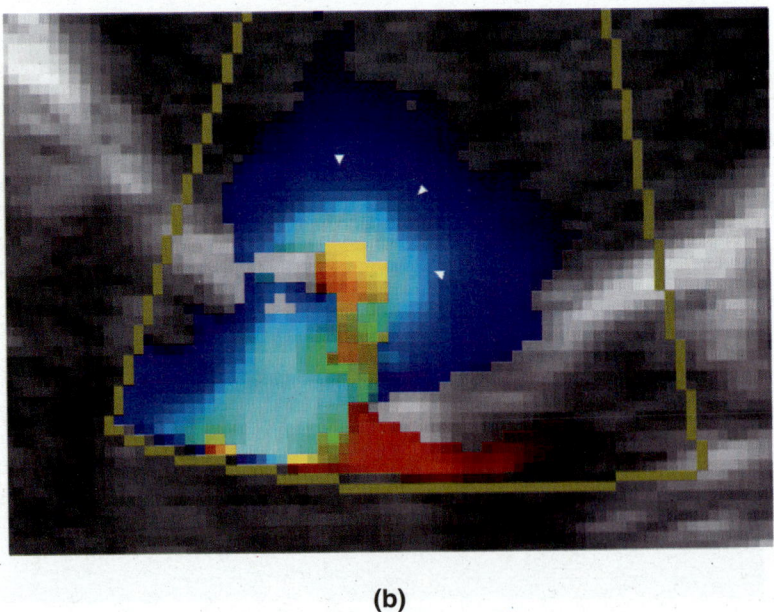

(b)

Figure 4.10 (a) Antegrade colour flow across the mitral valve in severe mitral stenosis. **(b)** Note the appearance of proximal iso-velocity area (PISA) shown by arrows in zoomed image. As the flow converges towards the stenotic valve there is aliasing since the velocity of blood flow exceeds the Nyquist limits. The area of hemisphere formed by this colour is calculated and multiplied by the velocity of blood to give the flow across the stenosed valve. This is used to quantify the severity of valve stenosis.

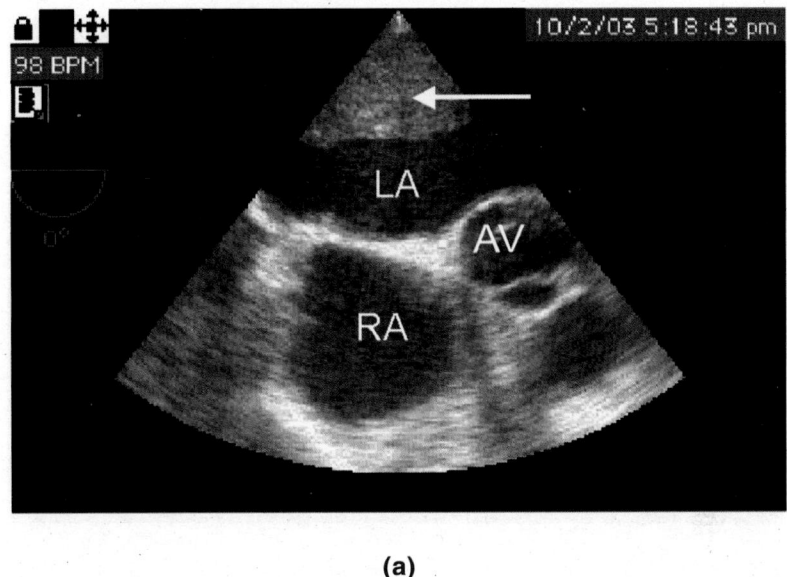

(a)

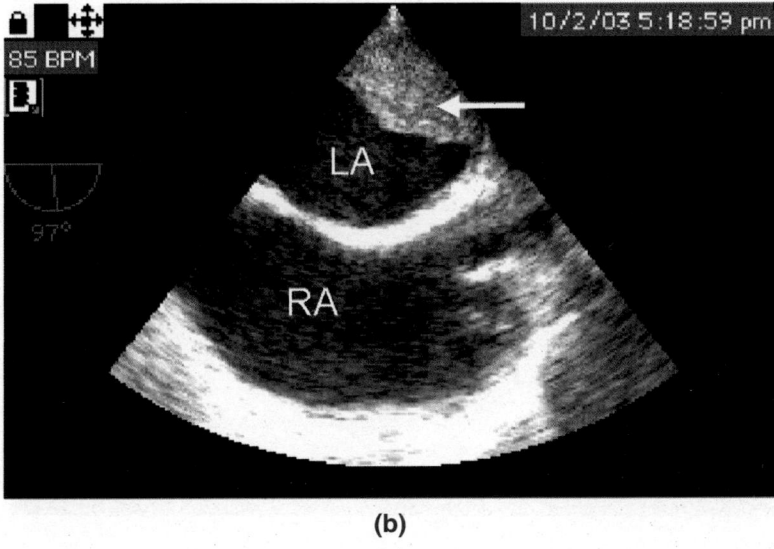

(b)

Figure 4.11. Large left atrial body clot (arrow) in a patient with severe mitral stenosis seen in short axis **(a)** and bicaval view **(b)** (LA: left atrium, RA: right atrium, AV: aortic valve)

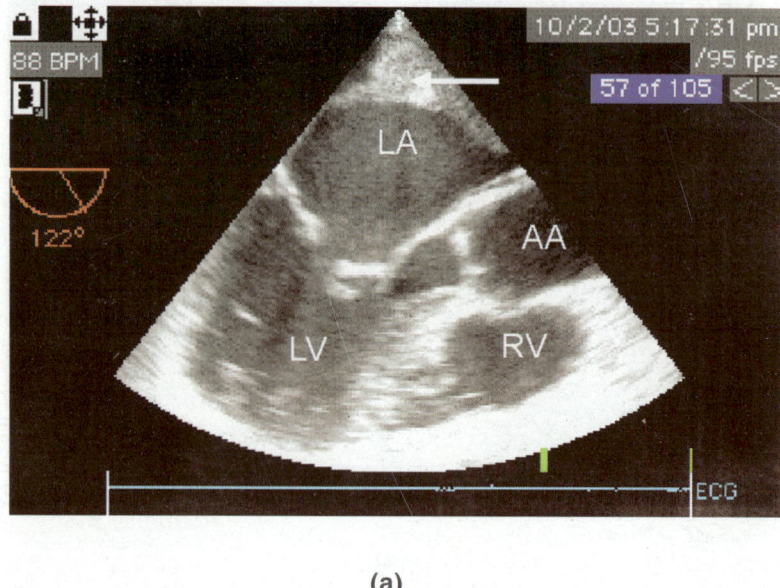

(a)

(b)

Figure 4.12 (a) Large left atrial body clot (arrow) in a patient with severe mitral stenosis layered across the posterior wall of the left atrium. **(b)** A mobile left atrial body clot (arrow) in another patient with mitral stenosis. (LA: left atrium, LV: left ventricle, RV: right ventricle, AA: ascending aorta, RA: right atrium)

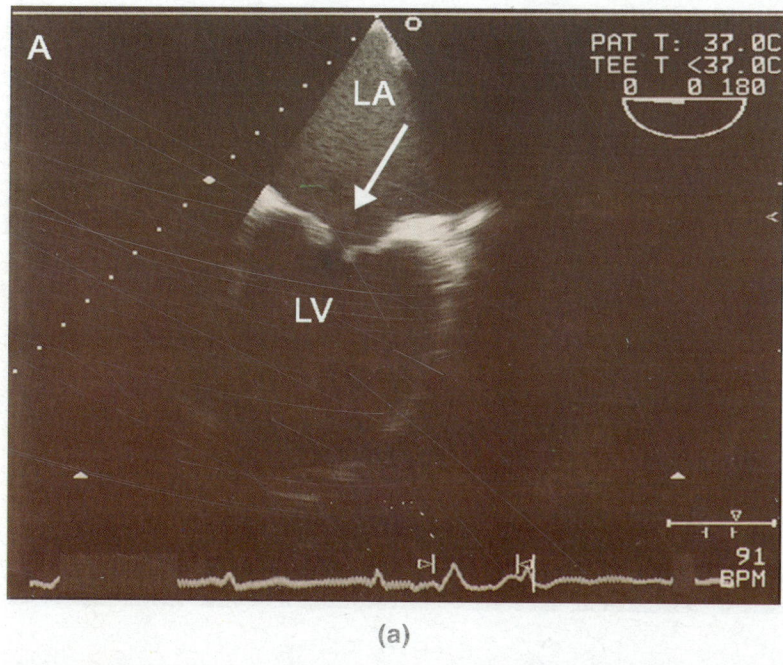

(a)

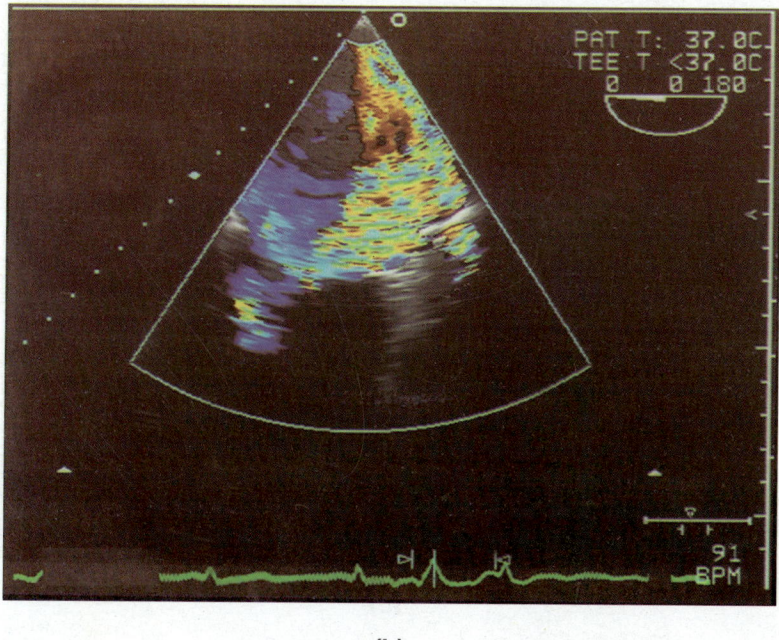

(b)

Figure 4.13 (a & b) Colour Doppler imaging showing severe mitral regurgitation due to incomplete coaptation of the mitral leaflets (arrow) in two chamber view. (LA: left atrium, LV: left ventricle)

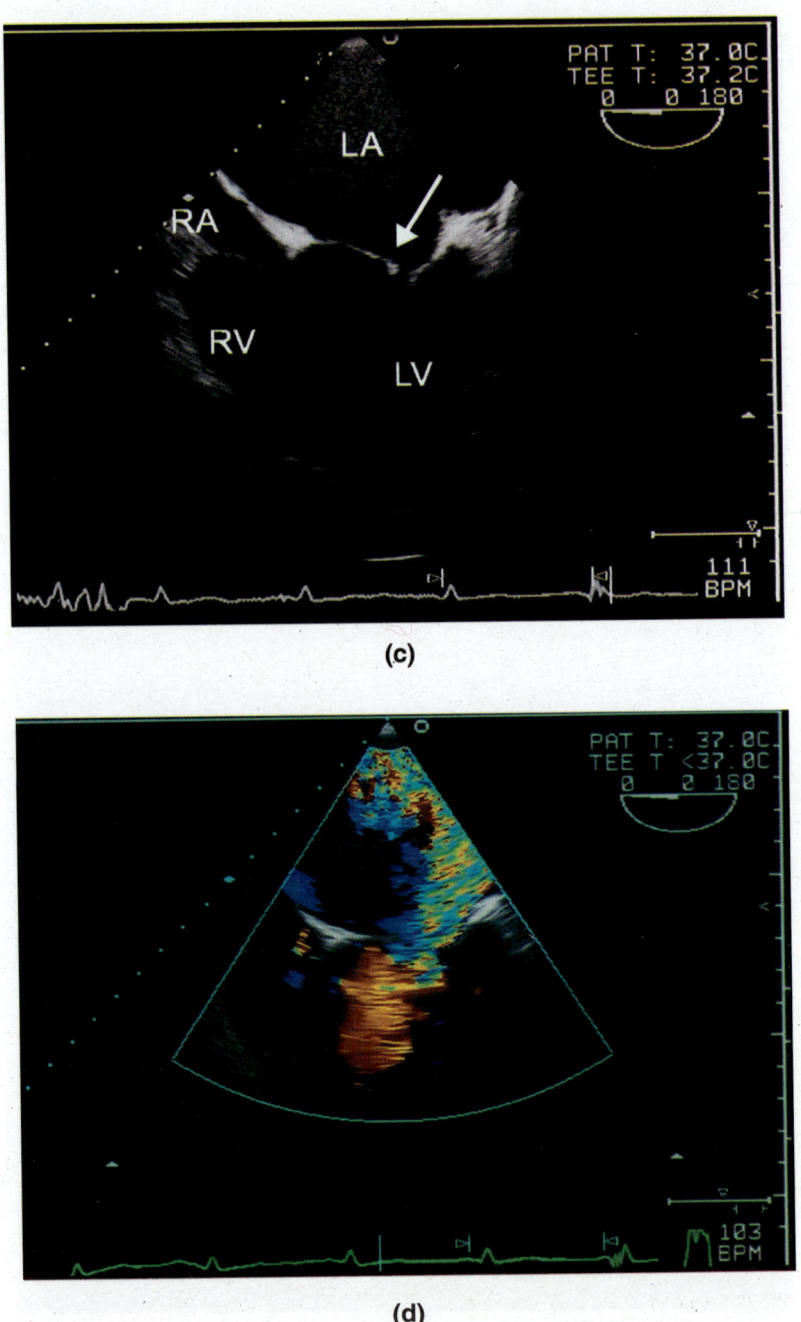

(c)

(d)

Figure 4.13 **(c & d)** Color Doppler imaging showing severe mitral regurgitation due to incomplete coaptation of mitral leaflets (arrow) in four chamber view (LA: left atrium, LV: left ventricle, RA: right atrium, RV: right ventricle)

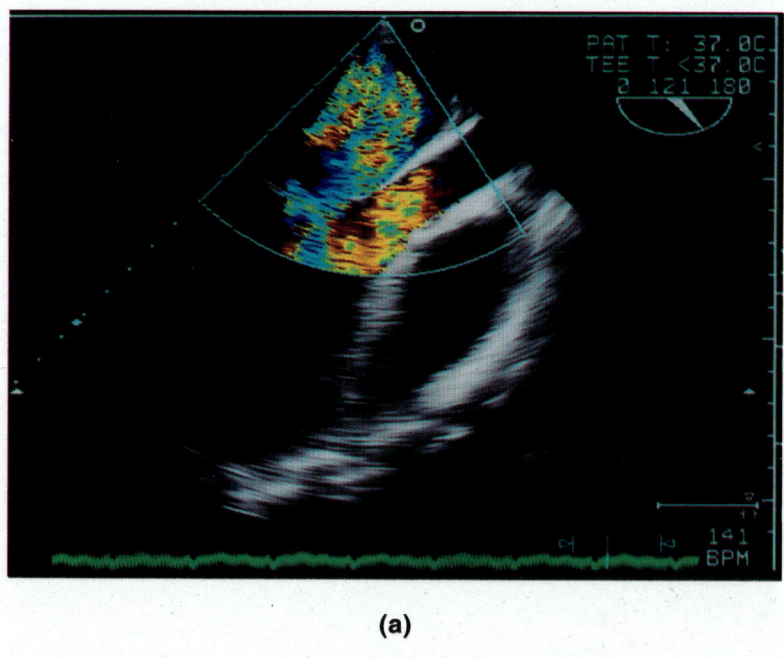

(a)

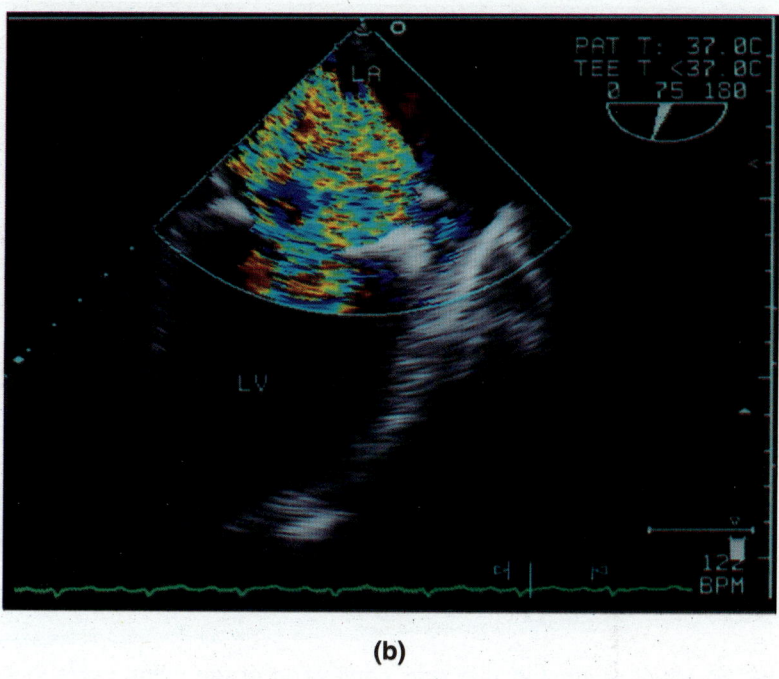

(b)

Figure 4.14. Appearance of severe mitral regurgitation on colour flow imaging in three chamber **(a)** and two chamber **(b)** views.

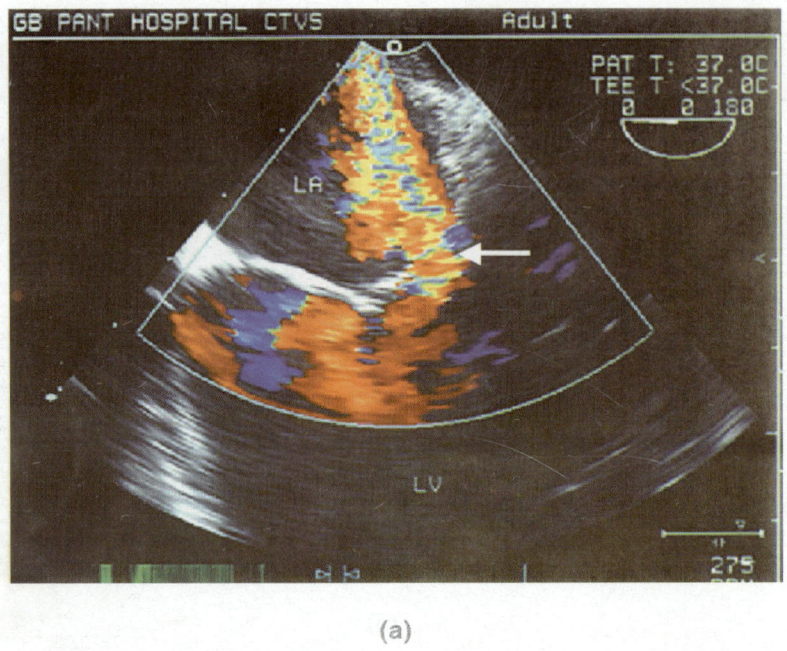

(a)

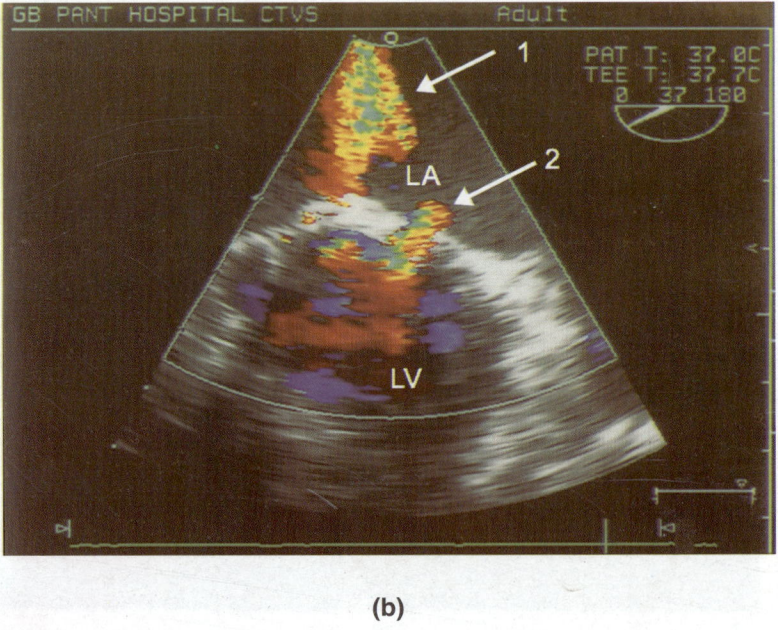

(b)

Figure 4.15 (a) Mitral regurgitation due to perforation of the mitral valve leaflet. Note the regurgitant orifice which is located at the base of the posterior mitral leaflet (arrow). **(b)** Shows the echo picture with two regurgitant orifices in the mitral valve leading to regurgitant jets (arrows 1 & 2). (LA : left atrium, LV : left ventricle)

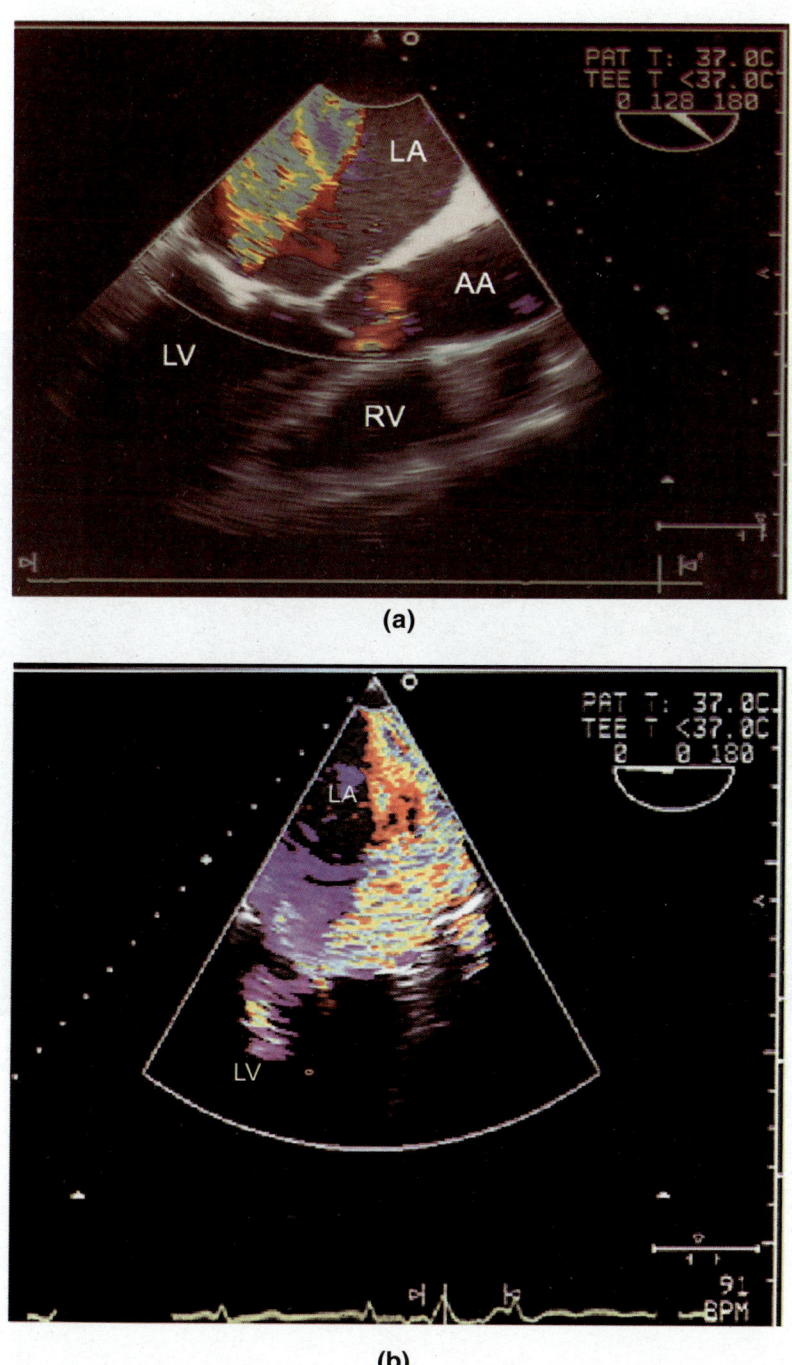

(a)

(b)

Figure 4.16. Appearance of mitral regurgitation (MR) on transoesophageal echo. **(a)** shows a central jet in a patient with moderate MR, while **(b)** shows an eccentric jet in another patient that is directed posteriorly. (LA: left atrium, LV: left ventricle, RV: right ventricle, AA: ascending aorta)

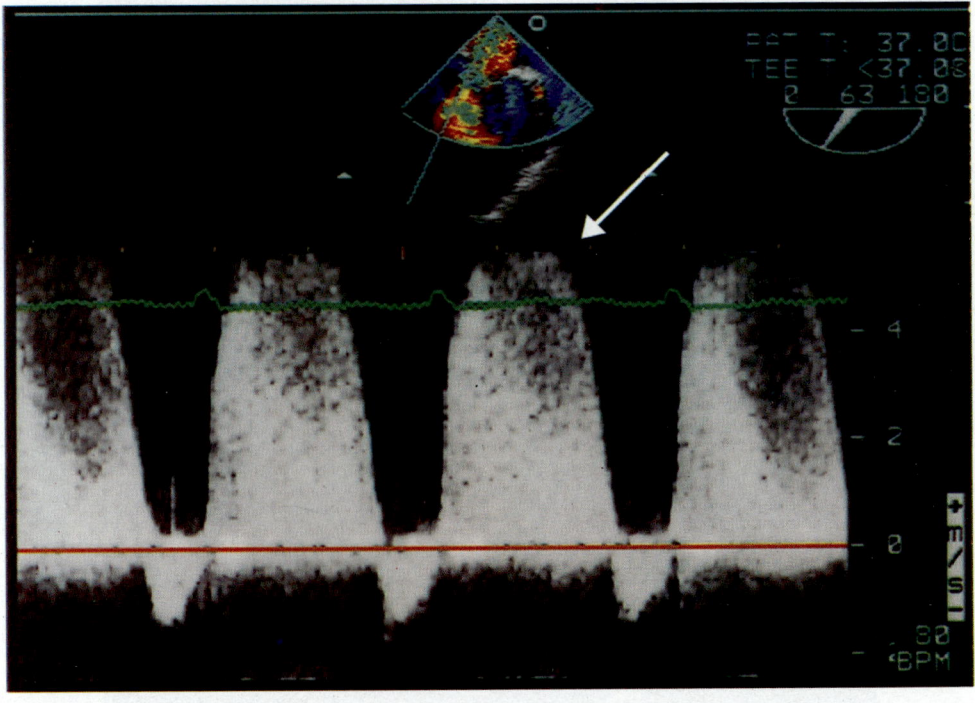

Figure 4.17. Continuous wave Doppler across the mitral valve in a patient with mitral regurgitation (MR). Note the high pressure spectral trace of MR (arrow).

Chapter 5

EVALUATION OF THE AORTIC VALVE

A careful and complete assessment of the aortic valve is a part of every transoesophageal echocardiographic (TOE) examination. The pre and post cardiopulmonary bypass assessment of the aortic valve in patients undergoing aortic valve replacement is useful to detect the adequacy of the valve function so that immediate surgical correction of paravalvular leaks can be carried out. The TOE examination of the aortic valve should include two dimensional images from multiple transducer locations and angles as well as colour flow Doppler displays.

The two main types of two dimensional views of the aortic valve are; short axis and long axis. In short axis views, the imaging plane is perpendicular to the direction of flow through the valve. This creates an image that appears as if you are looking directly at the valve from the ascending aorta. In long axis views, the aortic valve appears, as if you are looking at it from the side. The left ventricular outflow tract and the proximal ascending aorta are also visible. The deep transgastric view of the aortic valve is important as it makes the Doppler ultrasound beam parallel to the flow through the aortic valve (this is not possible from the midoesophageal views). This is useful for the calculation of gradients across the aortic valve and cardiac output. In this chapter all these images are illustrated along with the various possible abnormalities of the aortic valve.

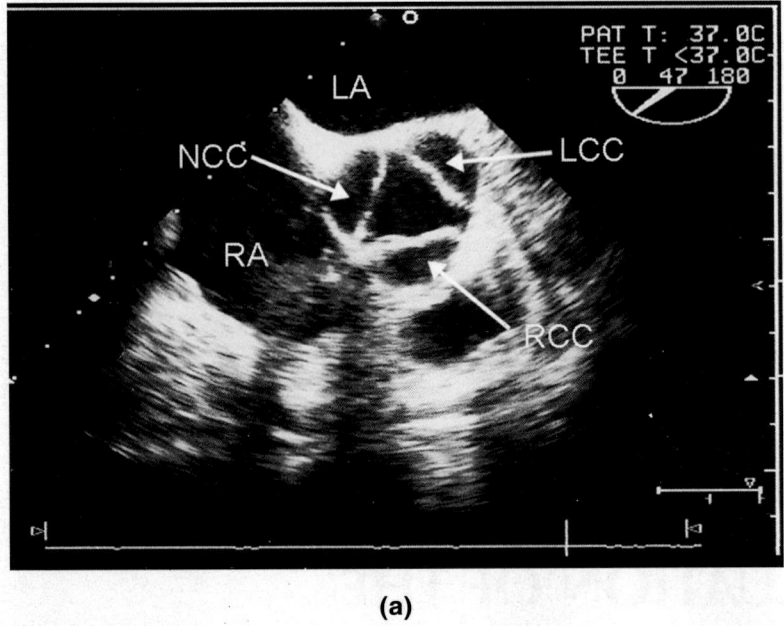

(a)

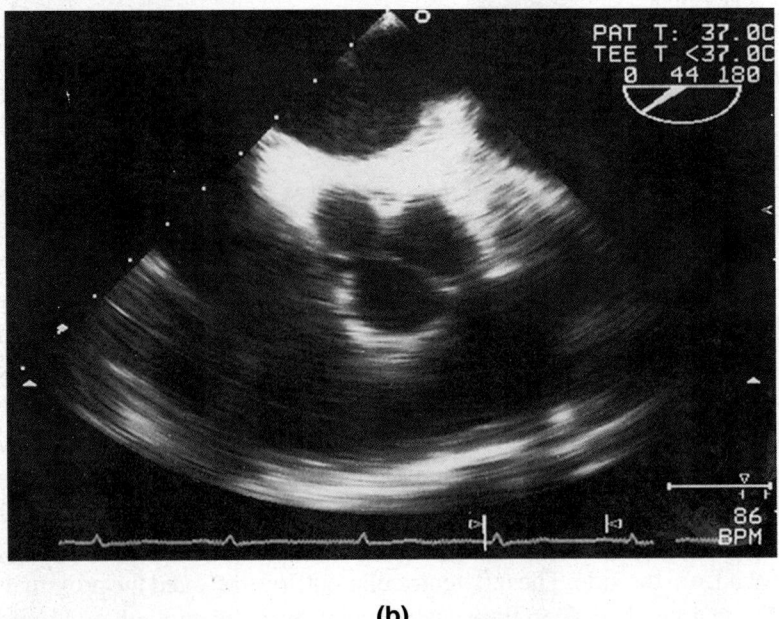

(b)

Figure 5.1. Short-axis views of the normal aortic valve in systole **(a)** and diastole **(b)**. (LA: left atrium, RA: right atrium, NCC: noncoronary cusp, LCC: left coronary cusp, RCC: right coronary cusp)

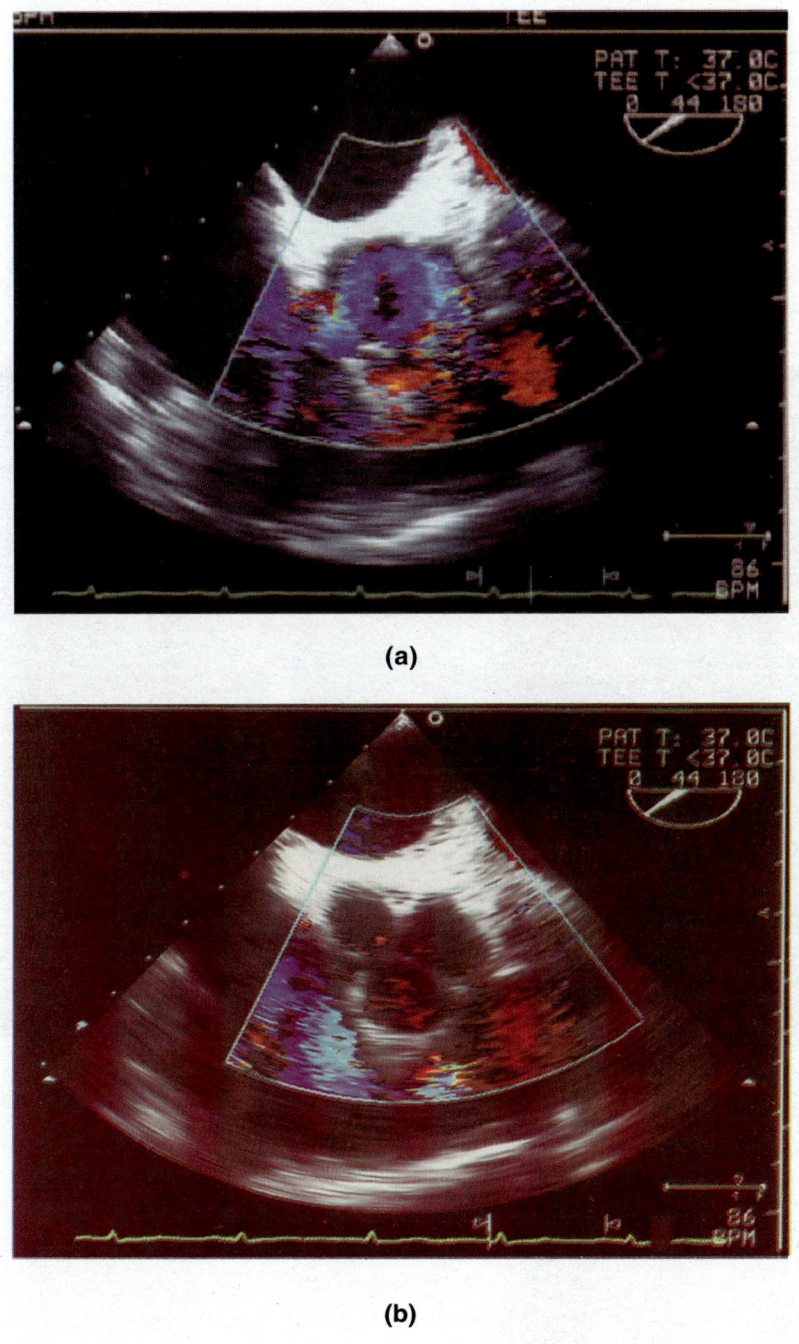

(a)

(b)

Figure 5.2. Colour flow across a normal aortic valve in systole **(a)** and diastole **(b)**.

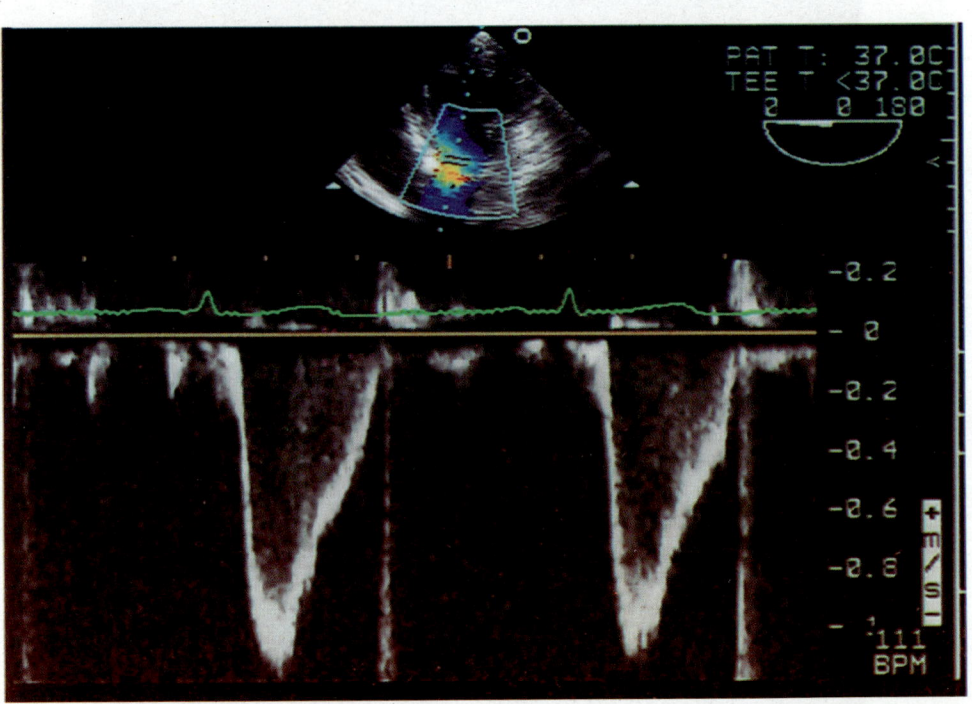

Figure 5.3. Pulsed Doppler flow across the normal aortic valve in deep trans-gastric view.

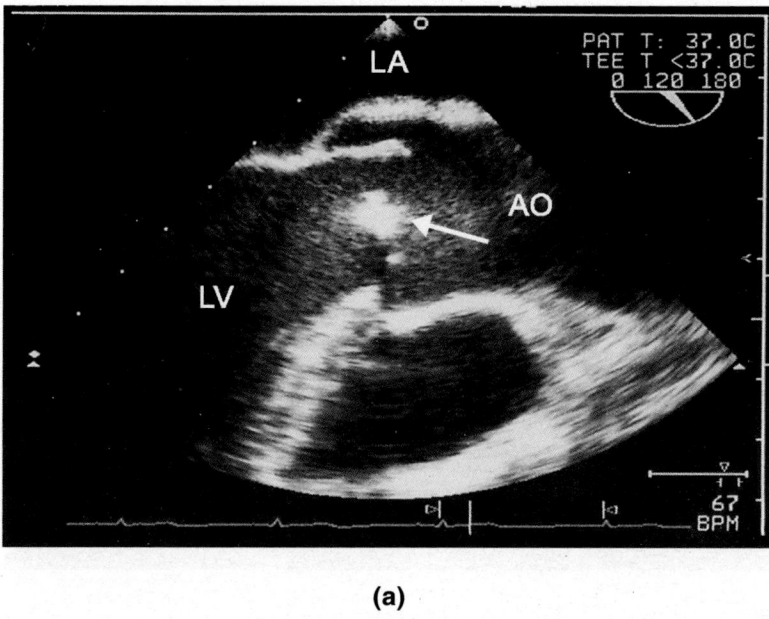

(a)

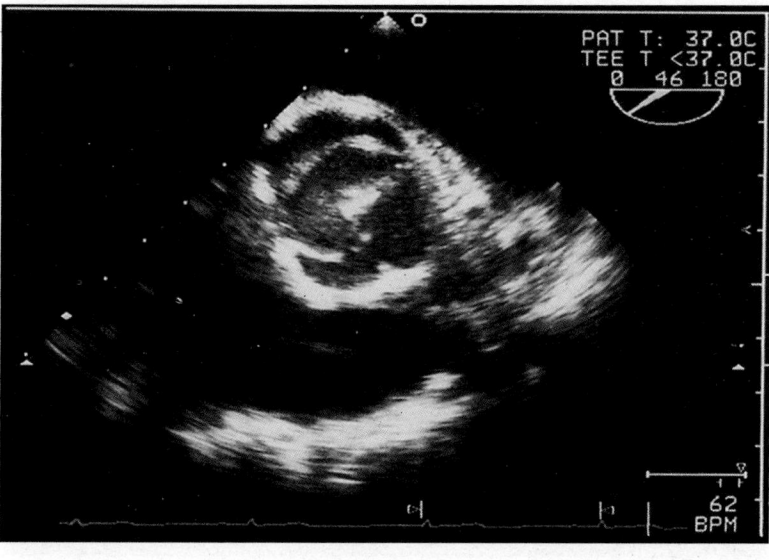

(b)

Figure 5.4. A patient with rheumatic aortic valve disease. Note the doming aortic valve in long axis **(a)** also note the calcific nodule on the aortic valve leaflet (arrow). Appearance of the stenosed aortic valve in short axis **(b)** This view can be used for performing aortic valve planimetry. (LA: left atrium, LV: left ventricle, AO: aorta)

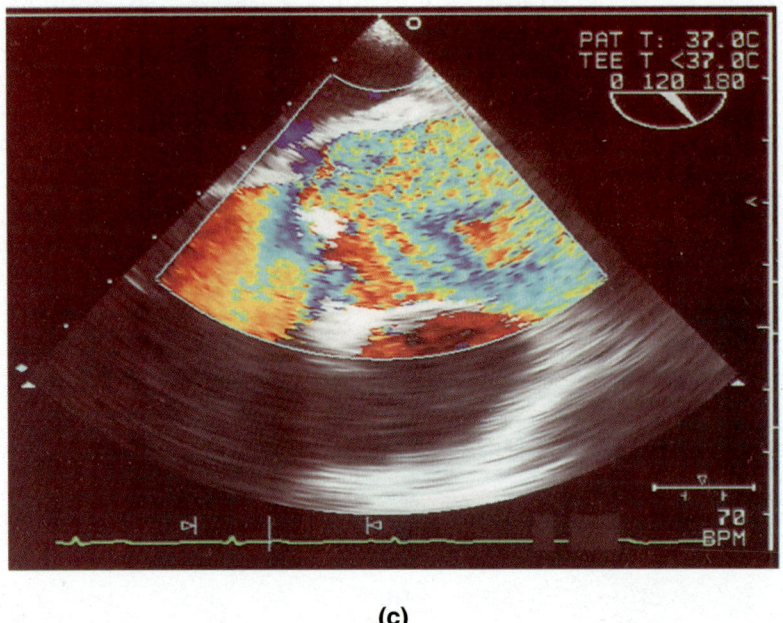

(c)

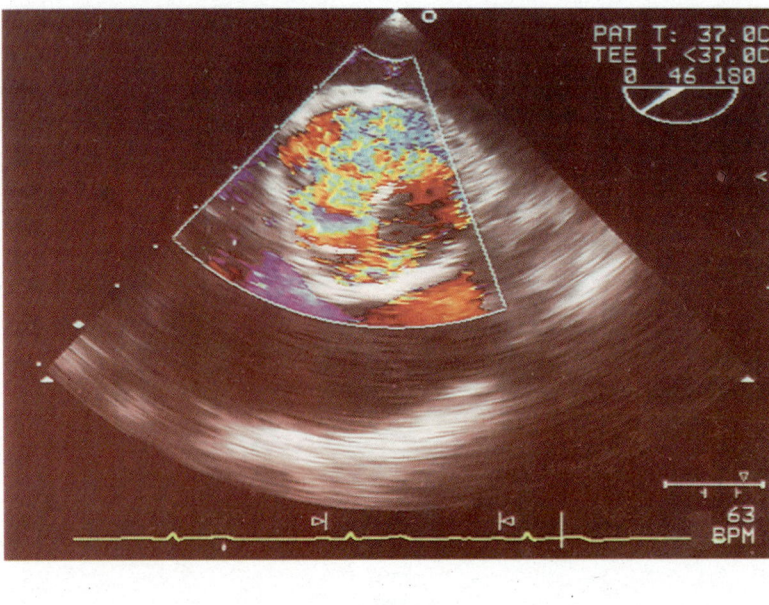

(d)

Figure 5.4. Systolic flow across the stenosed aortic valve in long axis **(c)** and short axis **(d)** revealing marked turbulence on colour flow.

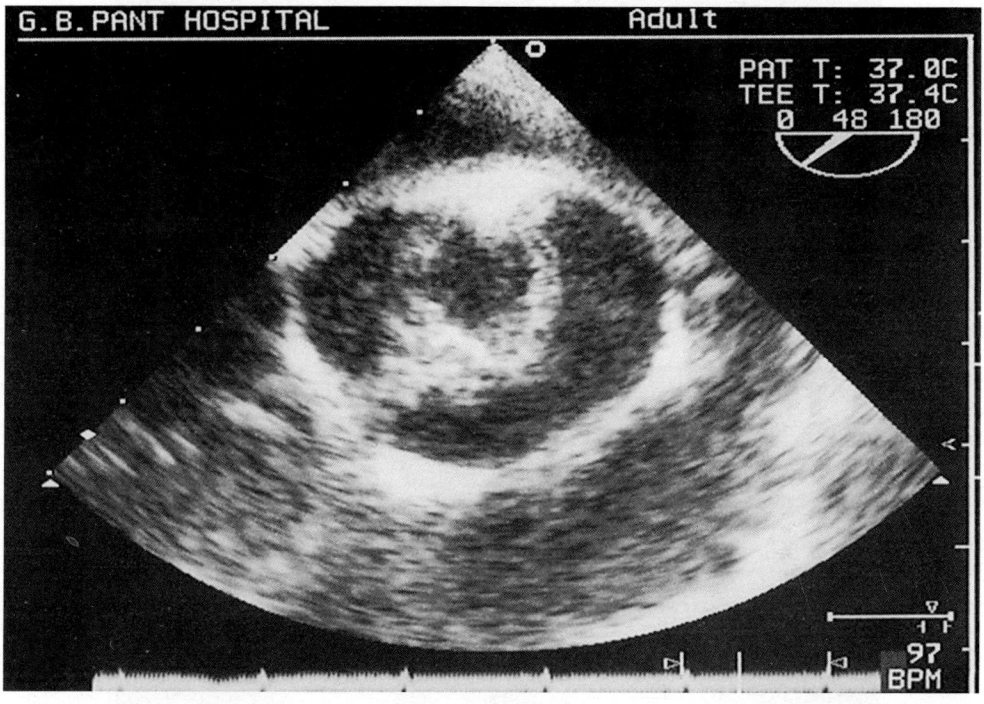

Figure 5.5. Appearance of a bicuspid aortic valve (short axis) with severe aortic stenosis.

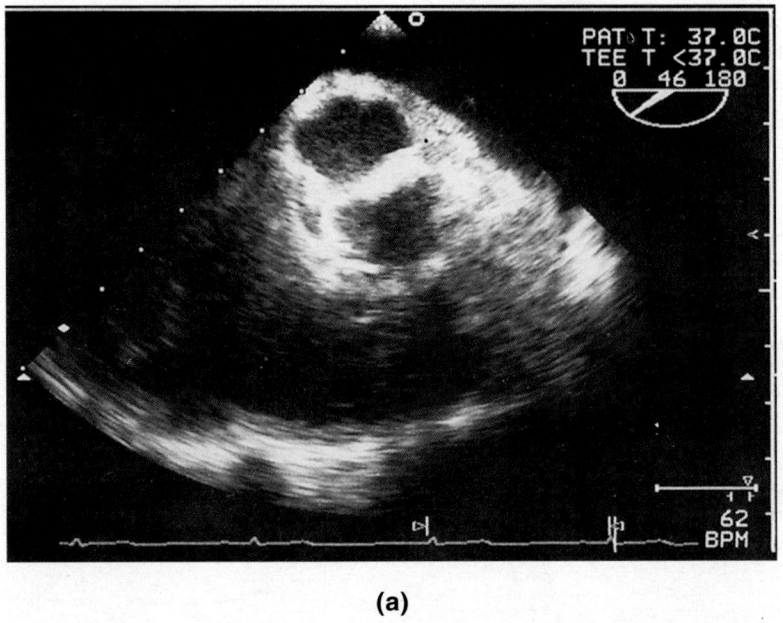

(a)

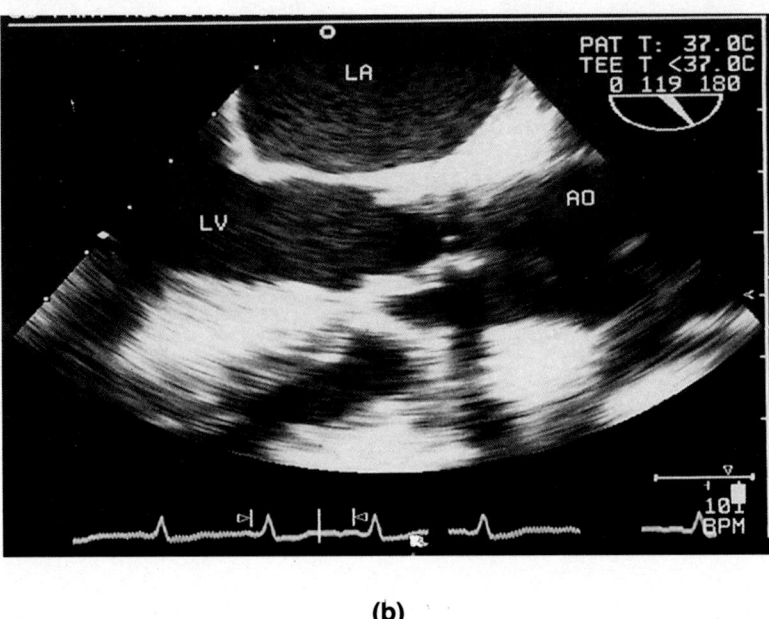

(b)

Figure 5.6. A patient with bicuspid aortic valve **(a)** Note the doming of stenosed aortic valve in long axis **(b)** (LA: left atrium, LV: left ventricle, AO: ascending aorta)

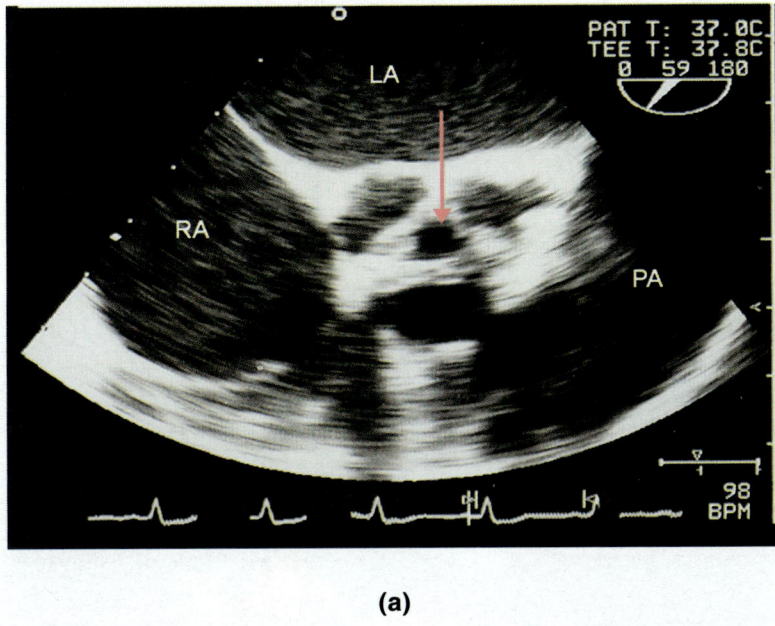

(a)

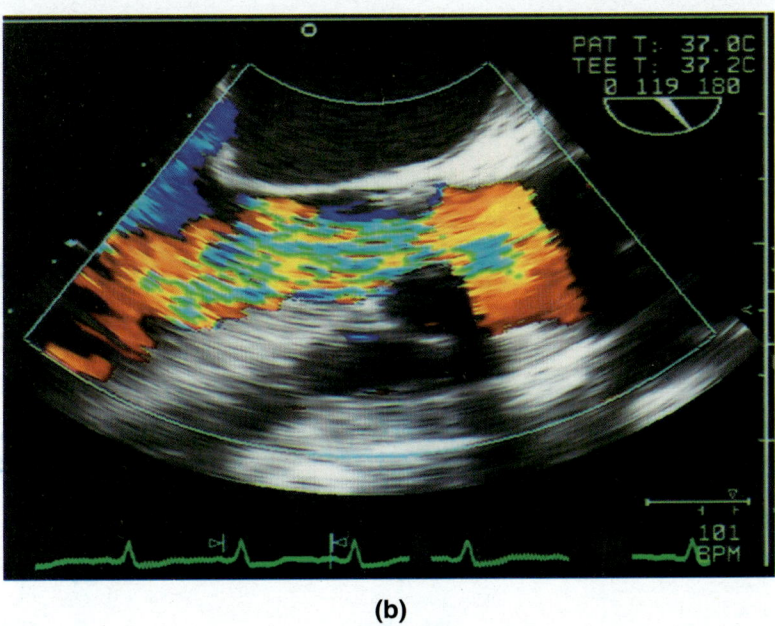

(b)

Figure 5.7. Appearance of the regurgitant orifice of the aortic valve in short axis (arrow) **(a)** in a patient with rheumatic aortic regurgitation. Note the colour flow across the aortic valve showing severe aortic regurgitation in long axis **(b)** (LA: left atrium, RA: right atrium, PA: pulmonary artery)

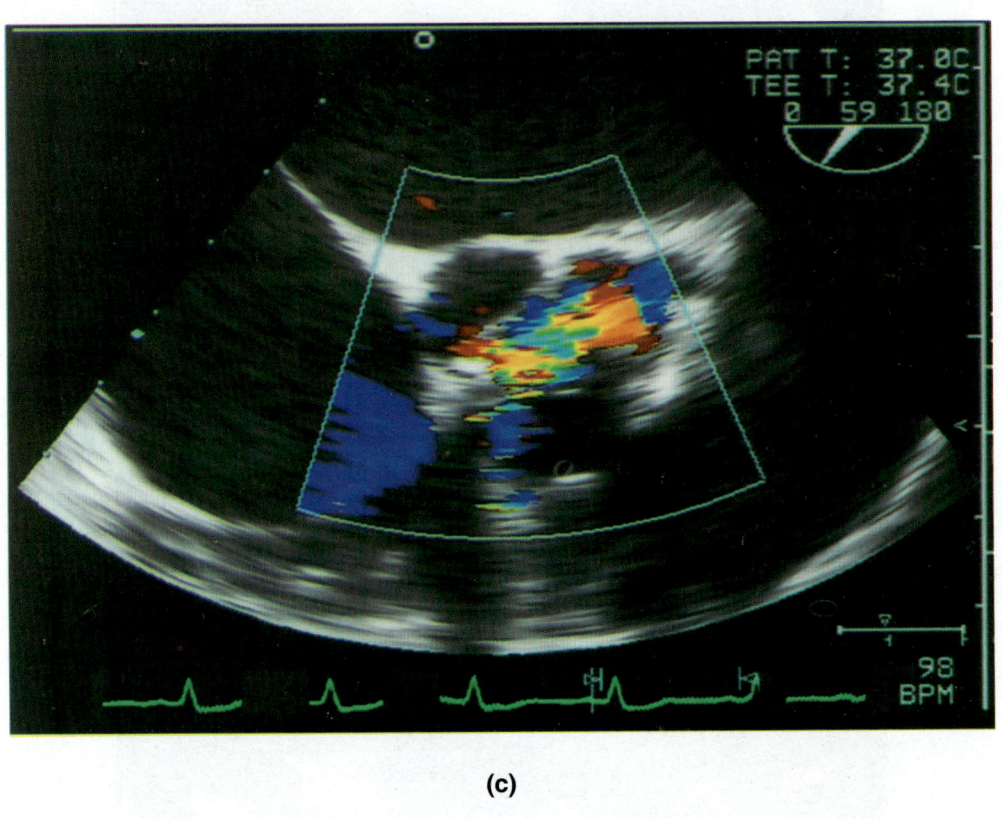

(c)

Figure 5.7 (c) Colour flow across aortic valve showing severe aortic regurgitation in short axis.

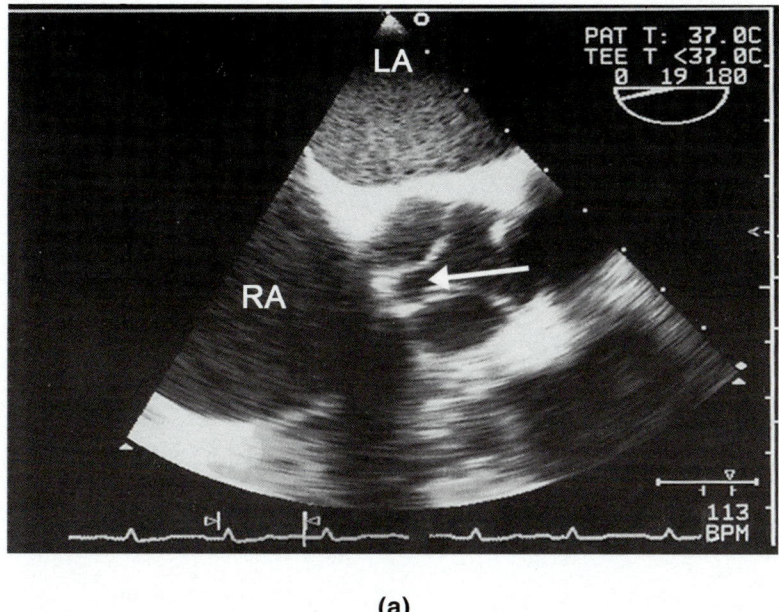

(a)

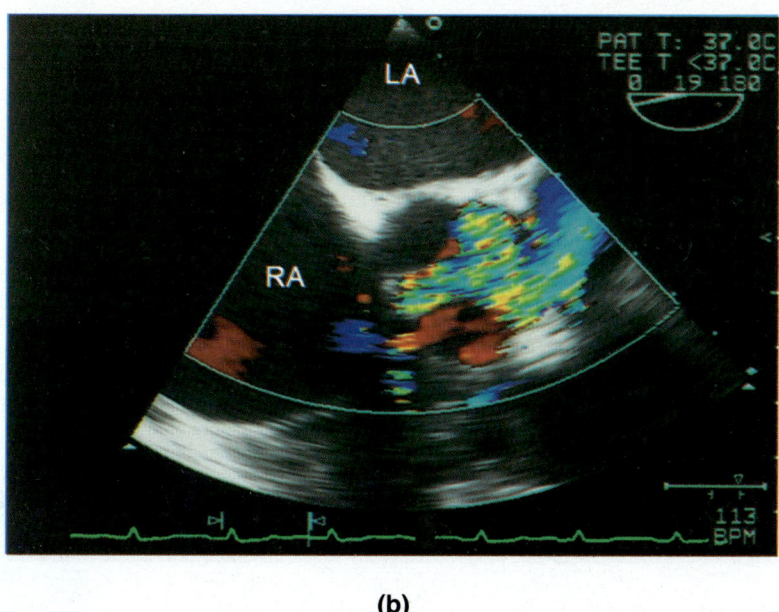

(b)

Figure 5.8. Incomplete coaptation of the aortic valve in short axis. Note the closed tricuspid leaflets **(a)** with a wide gap (arrow) in between. Colour flow across the aortic valve **(b)** in diastole showing the aortic regurgitation. (LA: left atrium, RA: right atrium)

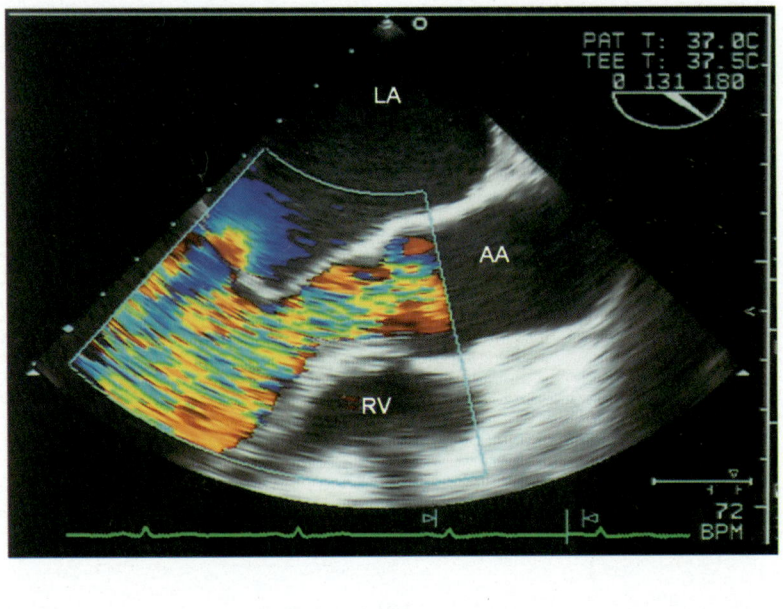

(a)

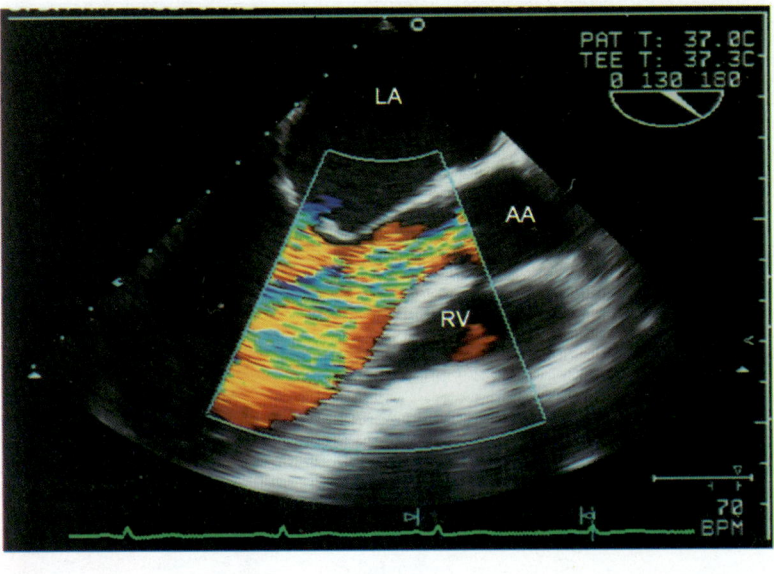

(b)

Figure 5.9 (a & b) Appearance of severe aortic regurgitation on colour flow mapping in two patients (LA: left atrium, AA: ascending aorta, RV: right ventride)

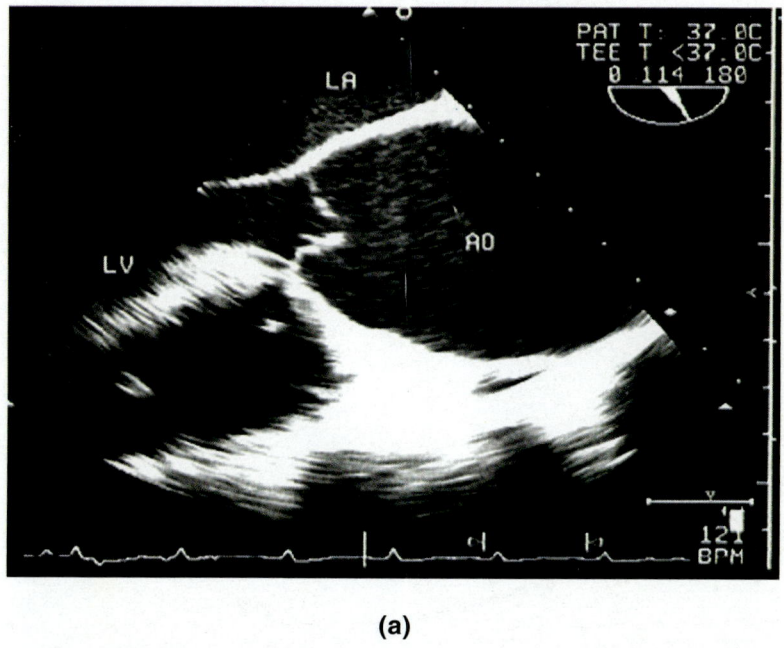

(a)

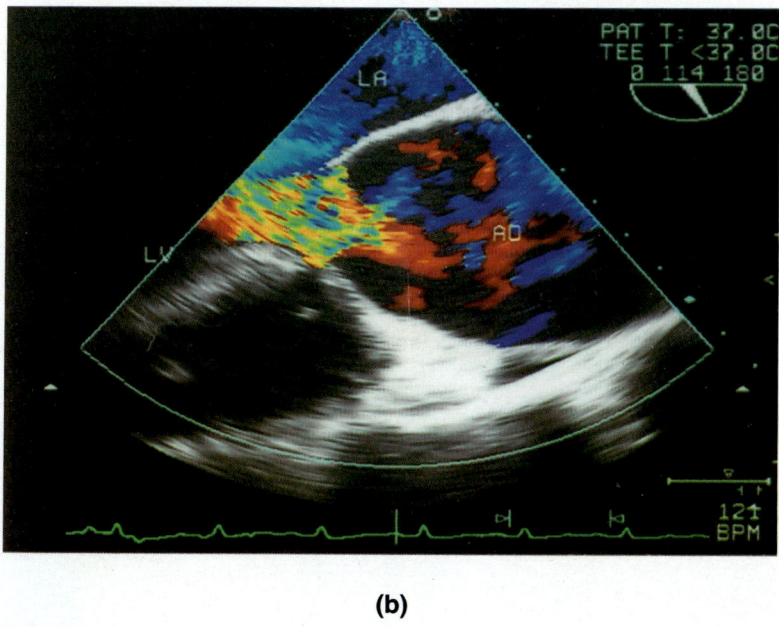

(b)

Figure 5.10. Dilated ascending aorta in a patient with Marfan's syndrome. Note the incomplete coaptation of the aortic leaflets and the incomplete closure of aortic valve **(a)** Colour flow across the valve **(b)** in early diastole showing severe aortic regurgitation. (LA: left atrium, LV: left ventricle, AO: ascending aorta)

Chapter 6

EVALUATION OF THE RIGHT SIDE OF THE HEART

The right side of the heart is perhaps the most neglected areas of assessment during trans-oesophageal echocardiography (TOE). The tricuspid valve, right ventricle and pulmonary valves can be accurately studied by TOE. In India, rheumatic heart disease is still common, so a large proportion of patients undergo valve surgery. Mitral valve surgery is the commonest operation in such patients. Assessment of the tricuspid valve is particularly important in these patients since tricuspid regurgitation is a common accompaniment in them. An accurate assessment of tricuspid regurgitation by TOE helps making a decision for carrying out tricuspid valve repair. Likewise, the assessment of the right ventricular function can guide the need for fluid requirements and pharmacological haemodynamic support.

Upper oesophageal views are used for the evaluation of pulmonary artery, four chamber and bicaval views for tricuspid valve and trans-gastric views for the right ventricle. In this chapter, the views demonstrating various possible abnormalities have been depicted.

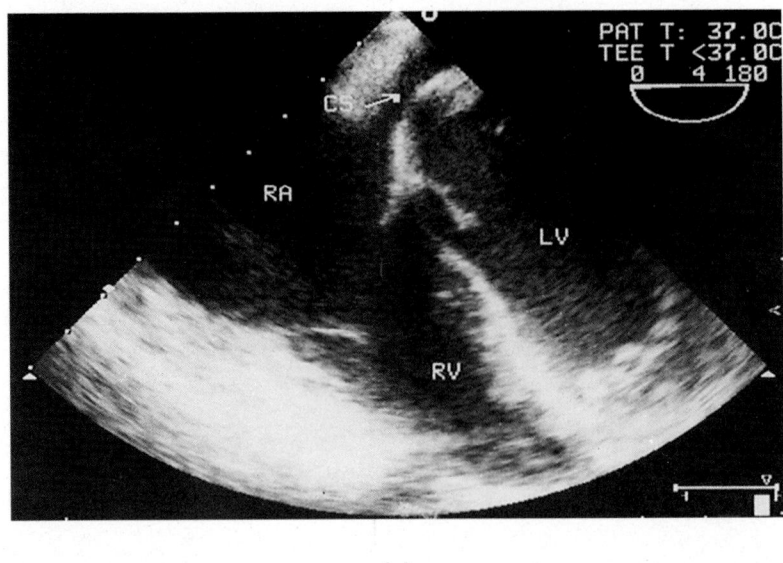

(a)

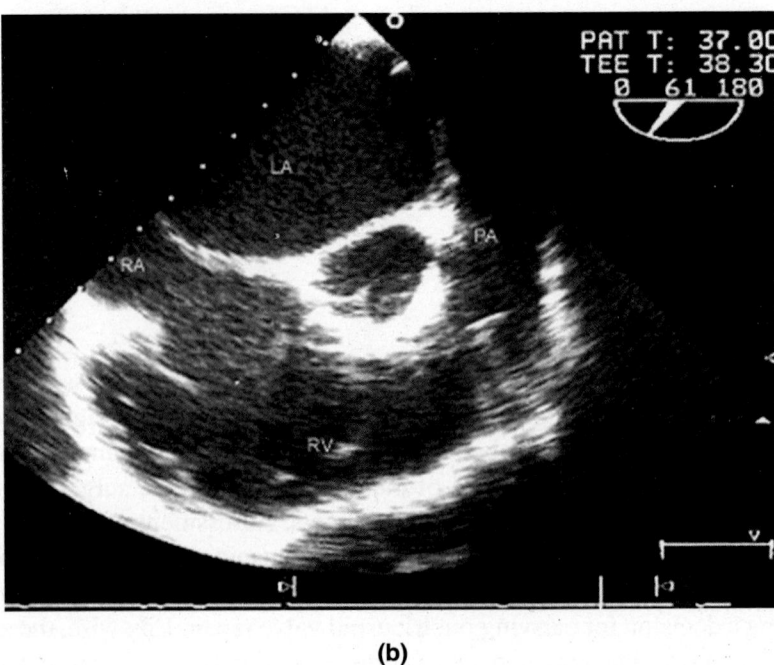

(b)

Figure 6.1. Modified four chamber view **(a)** and upper oesophageal view, 61° **(b)** for evaluation of the right ventricular function. Note the appearance of right ventricle in a normal individual. (RA: right atrium, RV: right ventricle, LV: left ventricle, CS: coronary sinus, LA: left atrium, PA: pulmonary artery)

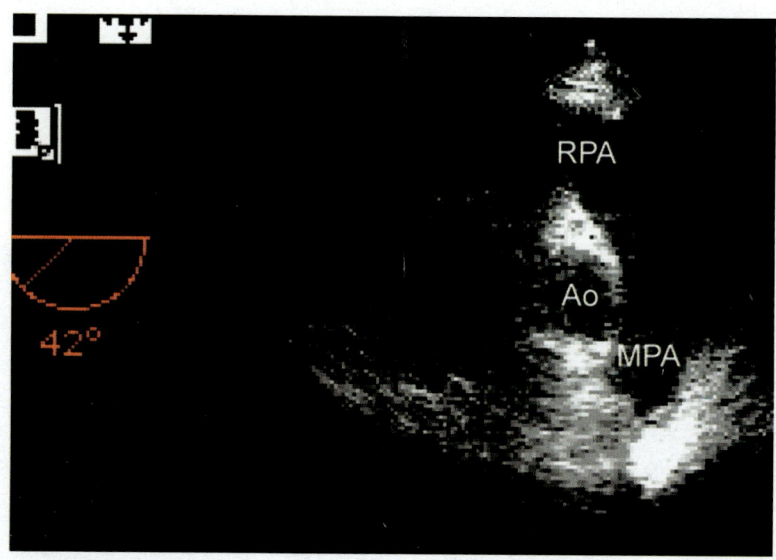

Figure 6.2. Upper oesophageal view for evaluating the main pulmonary artery and its branches. (RPA: right pulmonary artery, Ao: aorta, MPA: main pulmonary artery)

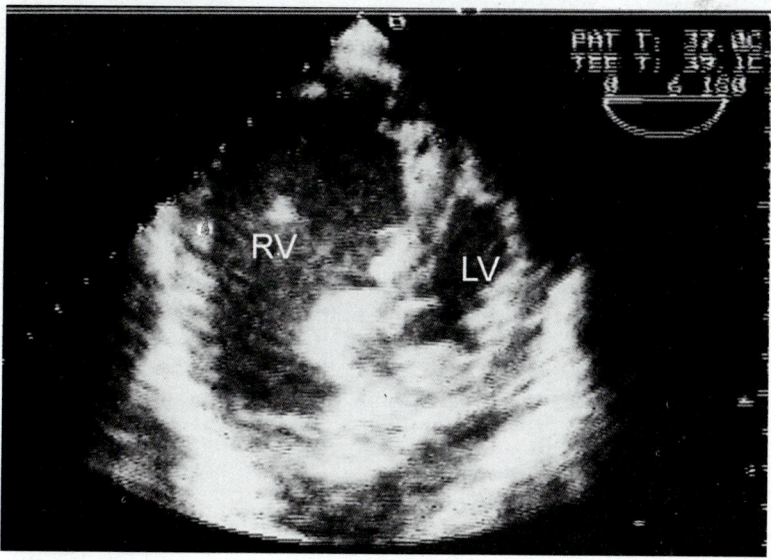

Figure 6.3. Deep trans-gastric view showing the ventricles in short axis in a patient with severe pulmonary artery hypertension and right ventricular (RV) dysfunction. Note the dilated RV and the deviated interventricular septum to the left. (RV: right ventricle, LV: left ventricle)

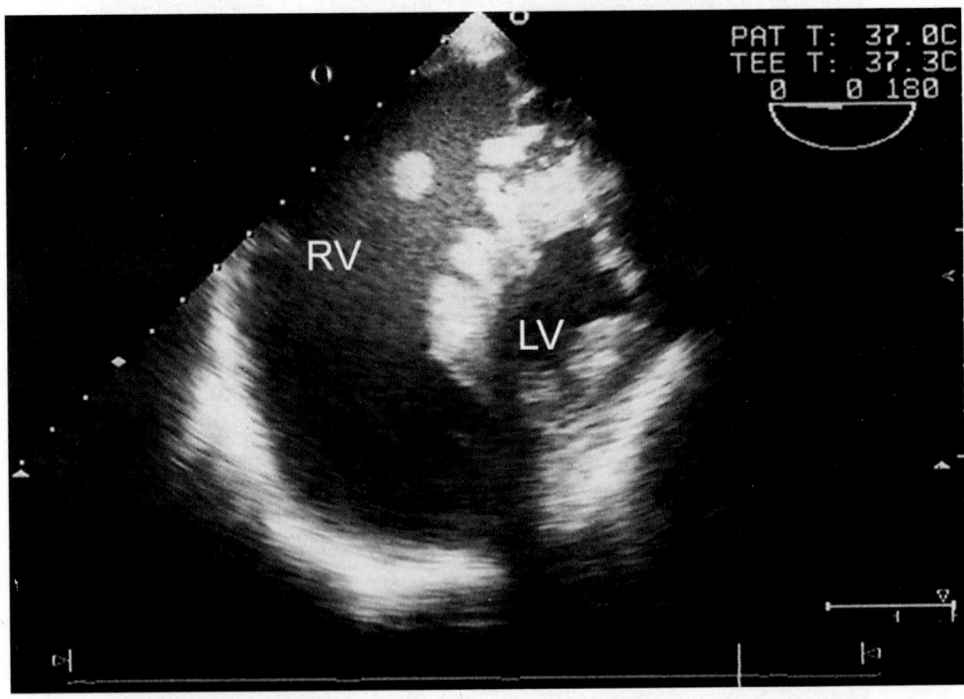

Figure 6.4. Transgastric view showing dilated right ventricle in a patient with a large right to left shunt (atrial septal defect). (RV: right ventricle, LV: left ventricle)

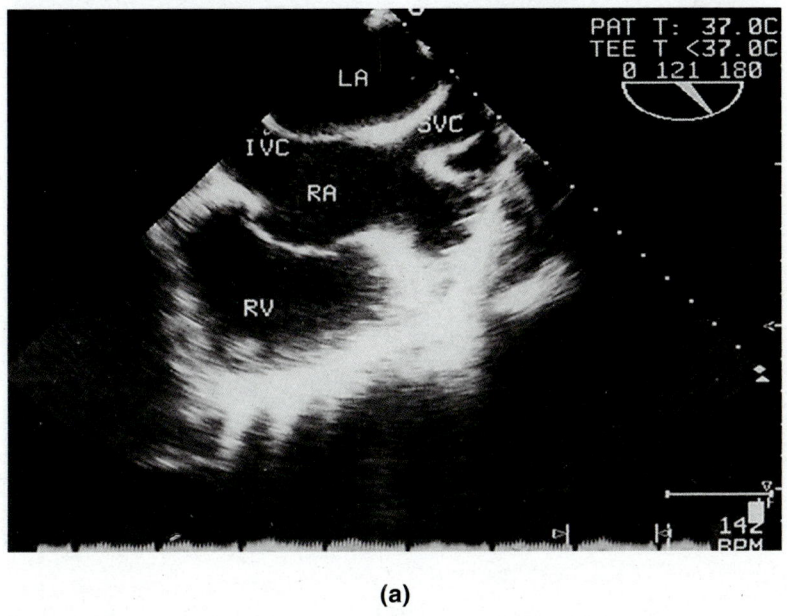

(a)

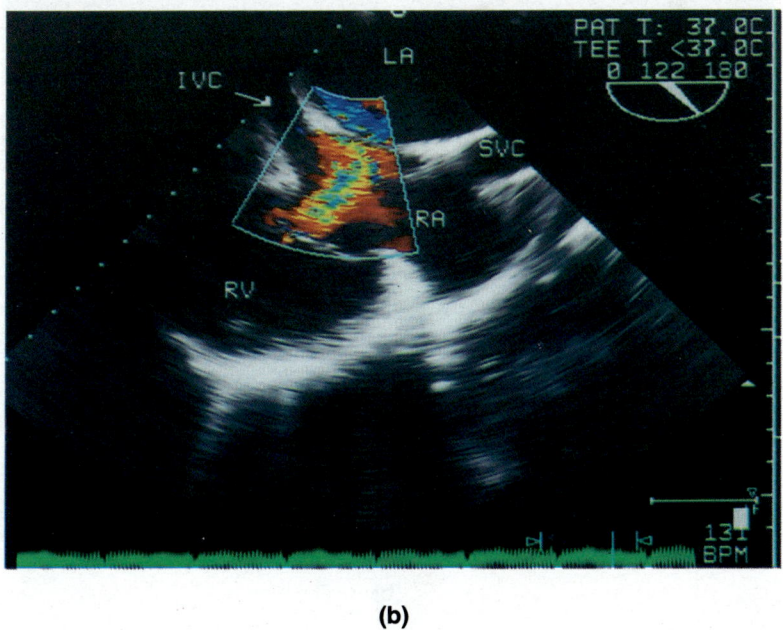

(b)

Figure 6.5. Appearance of the tricuspid valve **(a)** in bicaval view. Note the appearance of tricuspid regurgitation jet on colour flow study **(b)**. (LA: left atrium, RA: right atrium, SVC: superior vena cava, IVC: inferior vena cava, RV: right ventricle)

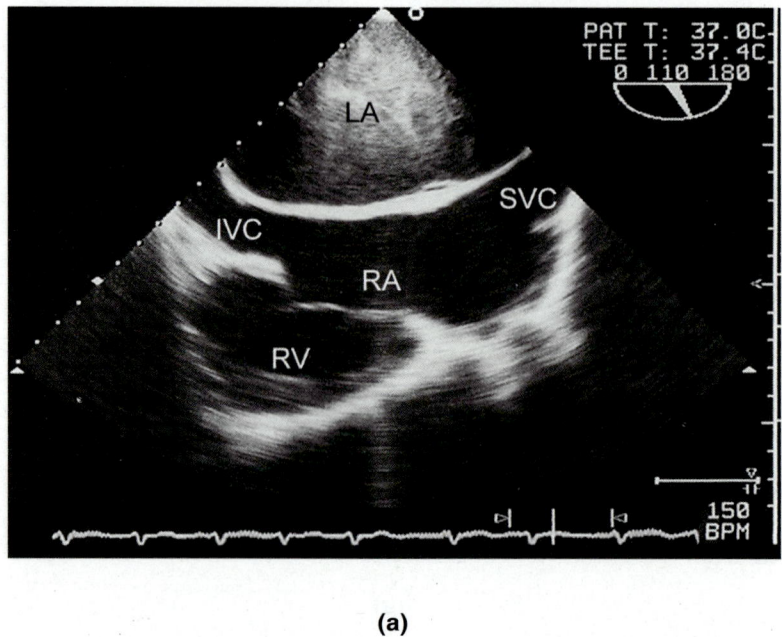

(a)

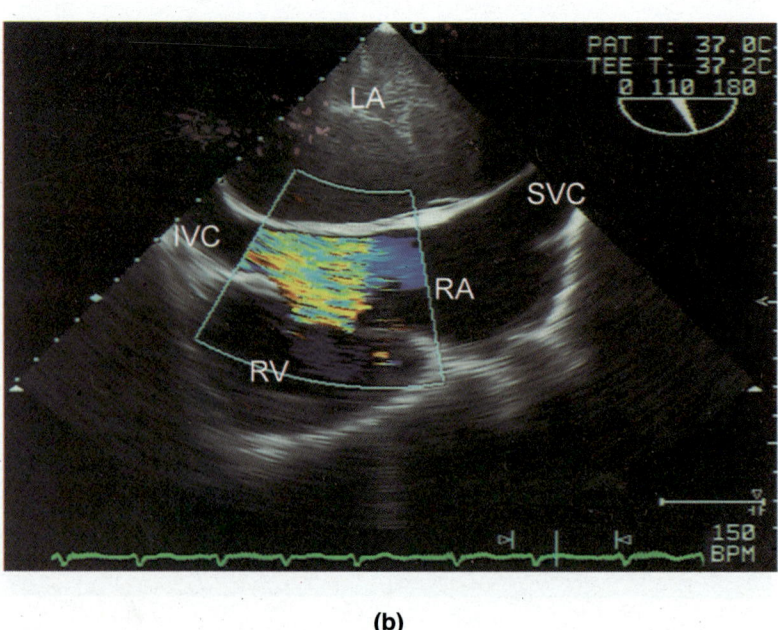

(b)

Figure 6.6 (a) Appearance of the tricuspid valve in a patient with rheumatic mitral stenosis (note the large left atrium with dense spontaneous echo contrast). **(b)** Shows the colour flow across the tricuspid valve showing severe hypertensive tricuspid regurgitation. (LA: left atrium, RA: right atrium, RV: right ventricle, SVC: superior vena cava, IVC: inferior vena cava)

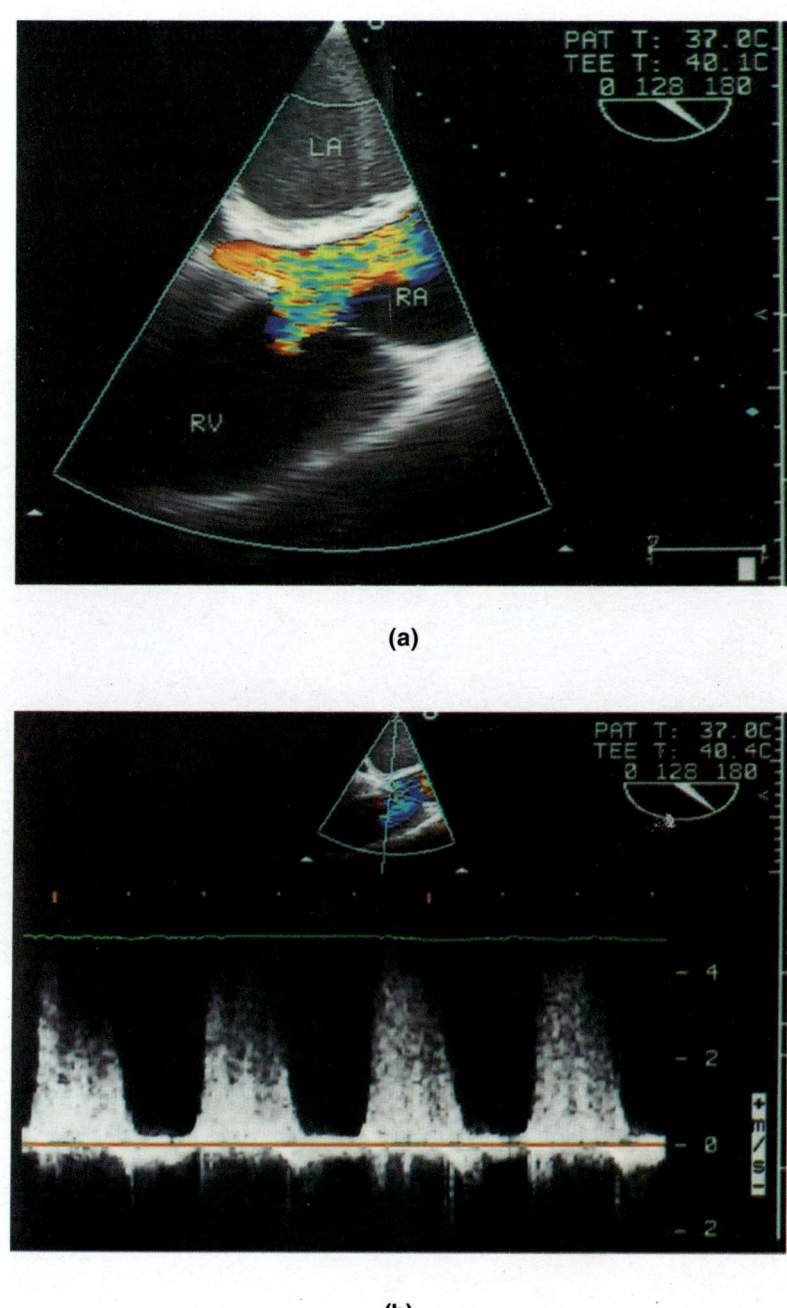

(a)

(b)

Figure 6.7 (a) Use of the bicaval view for proper alignment of the Doppler curser and the tricuspid regurgitation jet in a patient with rheumatic mitral valve disease and hypertensive tricuspid regurgitation. **(b)** Shows the flow velocity waveform. (LA: left atrium, RA: right atrium, RV: right ventricle)

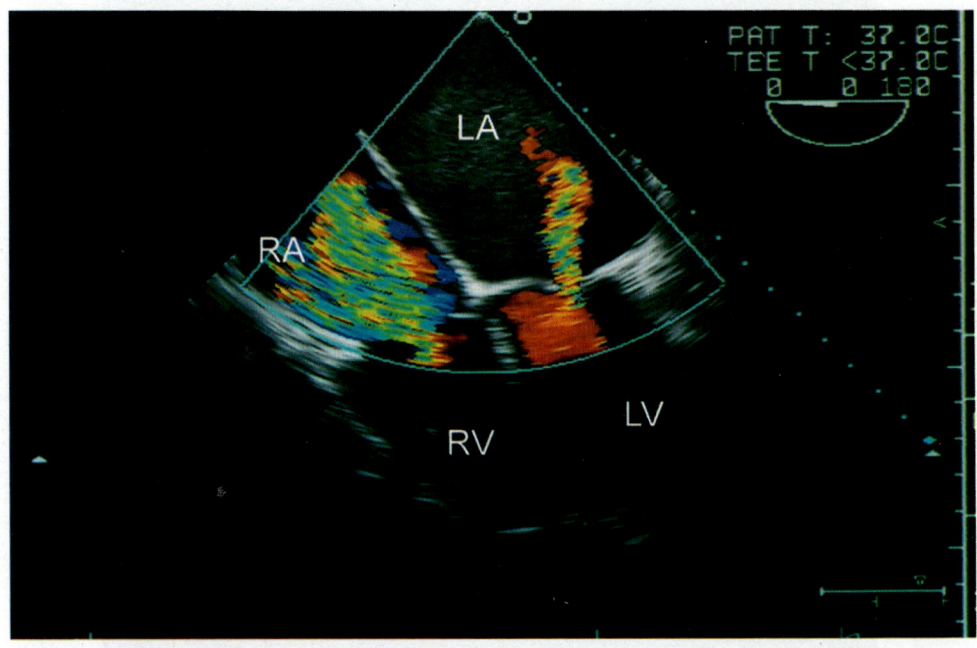

Figure 6.8. Appearance of severe hypertensive tricuspid regurgitation in a patient with rheumatic mitral valve disease. Note the enlarged left atrium with dense spontaneous echo contrast. Patient also has mild mitral regurgitation. (LA: left atrium, RA: right atrium, LV: left ventricle, RV: right ventricle)

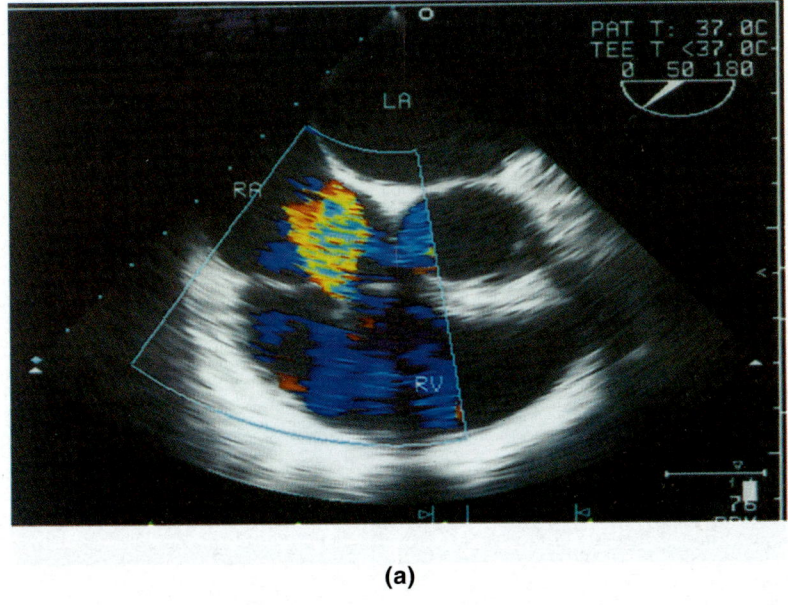

(a)

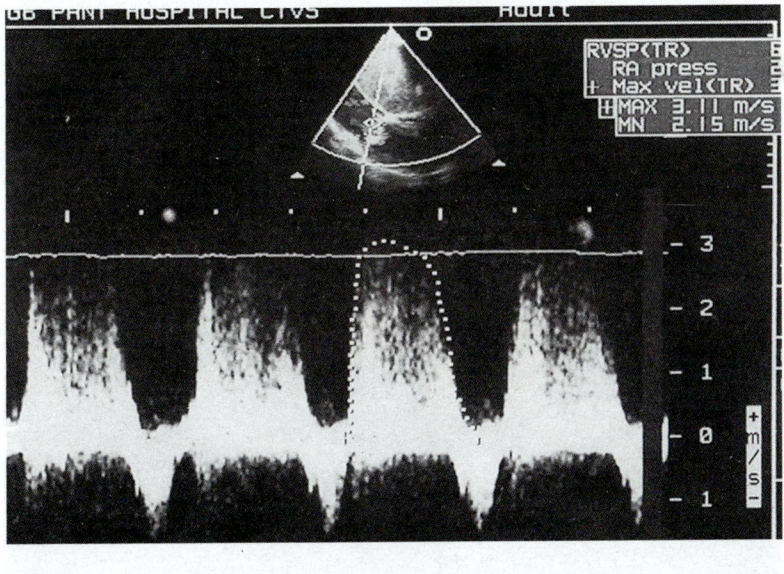

(b)

Figure 6.9 (a & b) Appearance of the tricuspid regurgitation in short axis view. Continuous wave Doppler can be used for estimating the right atrioventricular gradient (4 V^2 = 4 × 3^2 = 36 mm Hg). (LA: left atrium, RA: right atrium, RV: right ventricle, V: velocity)

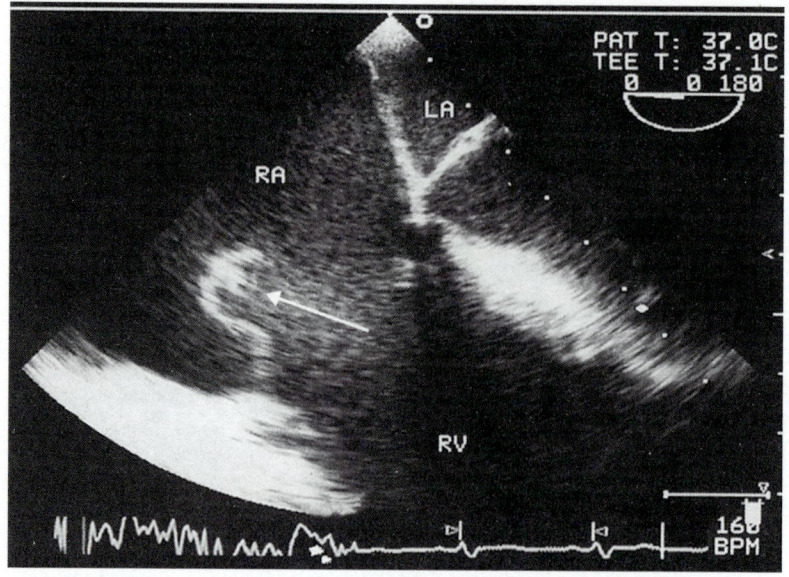

(a)

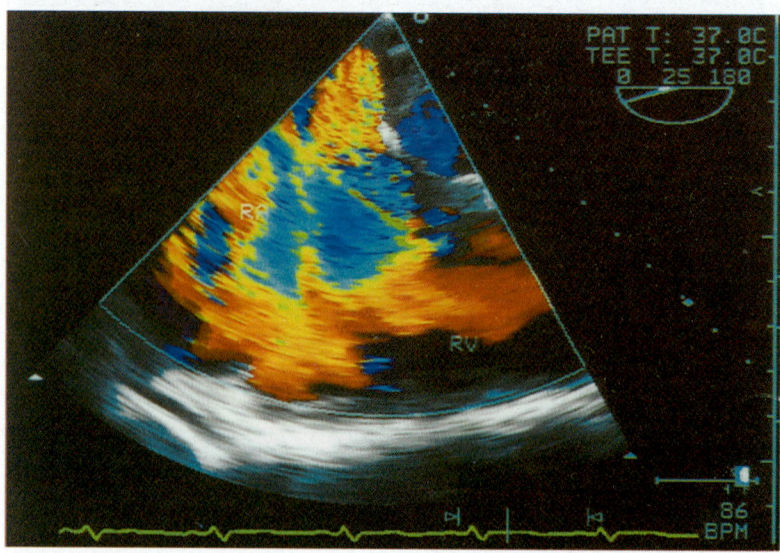

(b)

Figure 6.10 (a) A patient with congenital dysplastic tricuspid valve. Note the flail tricuspid leaflet (arrow). **(b)** The resultant severe normotensive tricuspid regurgitation on colour flow. (RA: right atrium, LA: left atrium, RV: right ventricle)

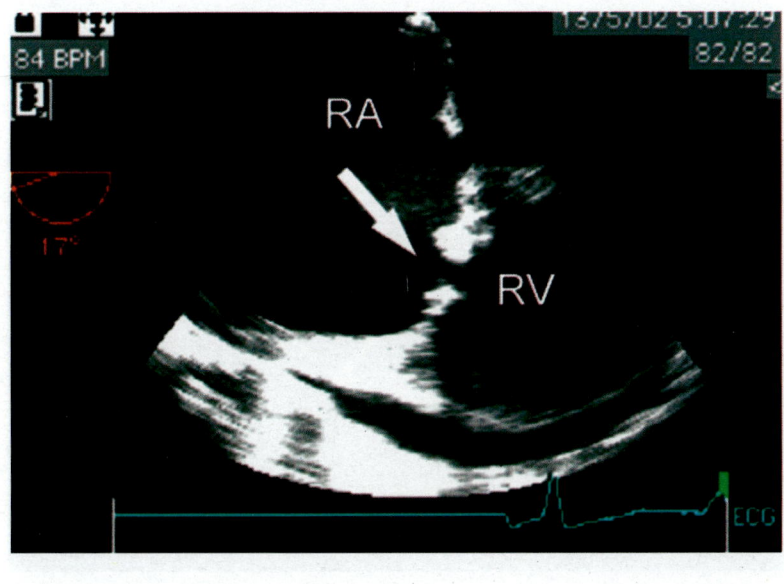

(a)

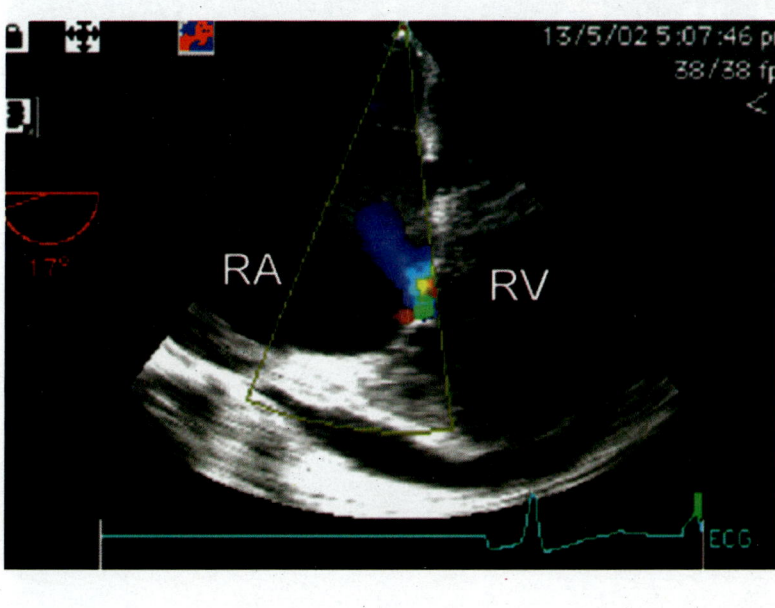

(b)

Figure 6.11 (a) Appearance of the tricuspid valve (arrow). Note the marked thickening, calcification and doming of tricuspid leaflets. **(b)** Colour flow across the tricuspid valve shows mild tricuspid regurgitation. (RA: right atrium, RV: right ventricle)

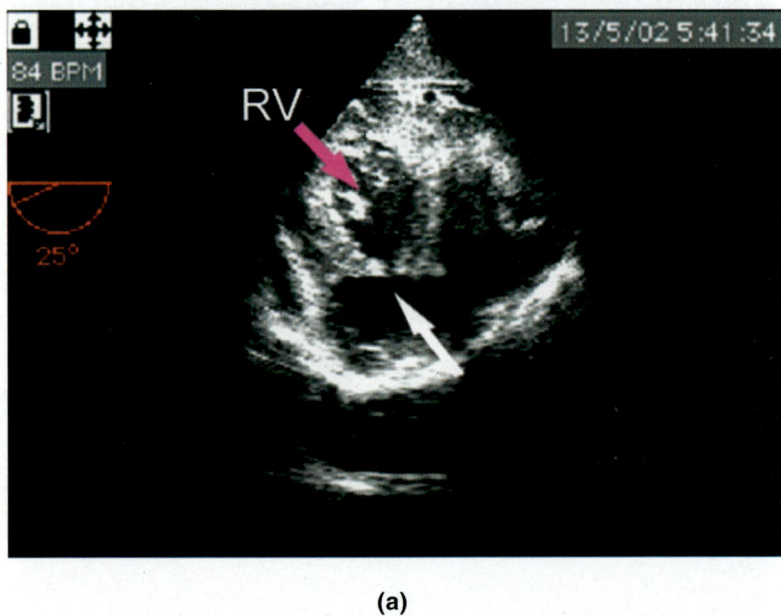

(a)

(b)

Figures 6.12 A patient with subpulmonary membrane.
(a & b) Appearance of sub-pulmonary membrane (arrow, **a**) in deep trans-gastric view of the right ventricular outflow tract. Colour flow (**b**) revealed marked turbulence caused by severe right ventricular outflow tract obstruction.

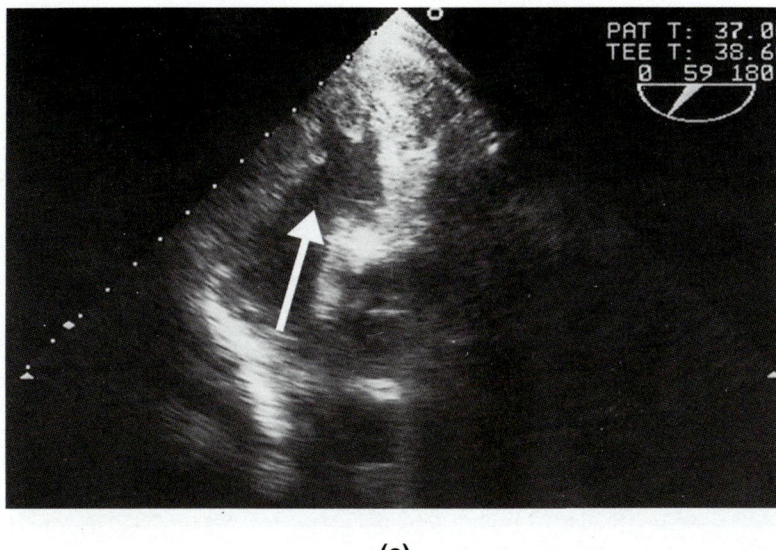

(c)

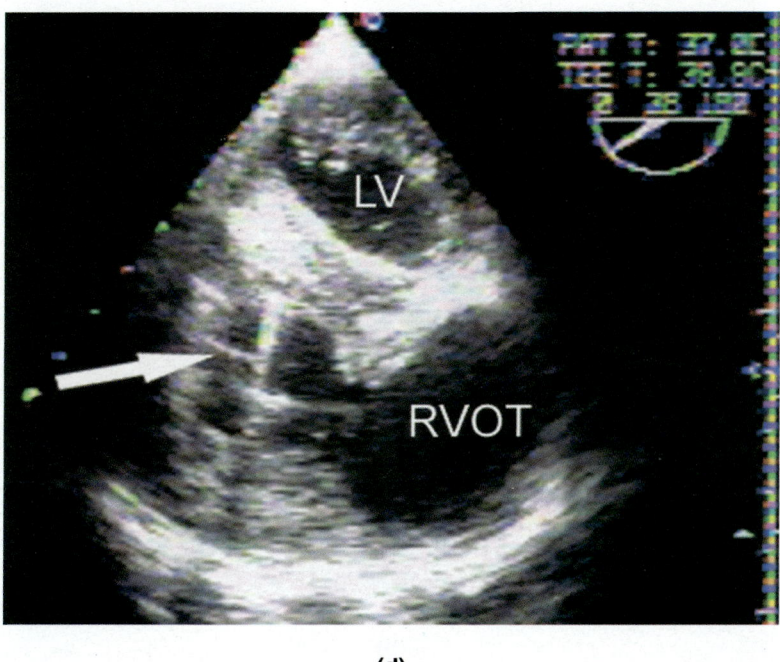

(d)

Figure 6.12 (c & d) Post operative appearance of the resected portion of the right ventricular outflow tract seen in deep trans-gastric view (arrow, **c**) and modified trans-gastric view showing Starr Edward prosthesis (arrow) in tricuspid position **(d).**

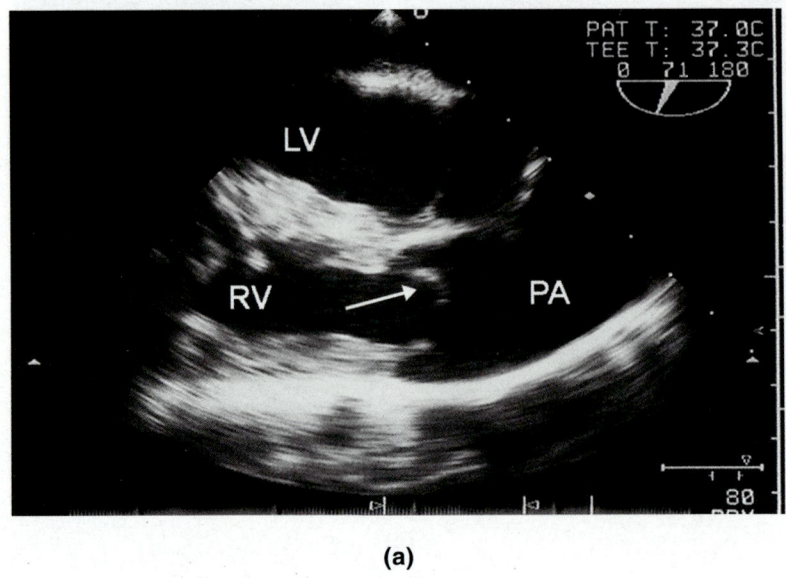

(a)

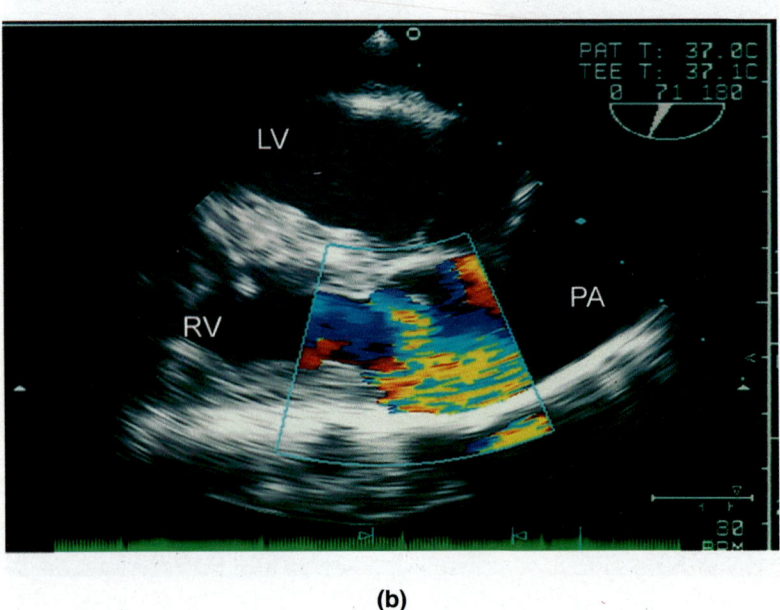

(b)

Figure 6.13. Appearance of congenital pulmonary valve stenosis. Note the doming pulmonary valve (arrow, **a**) and the turbulent stenotic jet across it on colour flow **(b).** (LV: left ventricle, RV: right ventricle, PA: pulmonary artery).

Chapter 7

EVALUATION OF THE PROSTHETIC VALVE FUNCTION

Assessment of the prosthetic valve function is one of the most important applications of transoesophageal echocardiography (TOE). However, evaluation of prosthetic valves can be complex, especially due to the fact that a large variety and different sizes of valves are available, each one of which has unique flow characteristics. Nevertheless, the functional assessment of a newly implanted prosthetic valve during surgery can be effectively performed in most patients. The metallic echodense components of mechanical prosthetic valves and the sewing ring and stents of bioprosthetic valves generate acoustic artefacts that may interfere with the visualisation of the prosthetic valve structure. In addition, these structures cast acoustic shadows, which interfere with the visualisation of structures on the side of the prosthesis facing away from the ultrasound transducer. For the same reason the blood flow on the side of the prosthesis that is facing away from the ultrasound transducer is masked, thereby interfering with the Doppler interrogation. As the transoesophageal probe lies directly posterior to the left atrium, the left atrial aspect of the prosthetic mitral valve is clearly visualised. Such an unobstructed view is not readily achieved with transthoracic probes. However, for evaluation of the ventricular side of a mitral valve prosthesis, trans-thoracic echo can be helpful. TOE is utilised for the assessment of the paravalvular leaks, which might necessitate reinstitution of the cardiopulmonary bypass and carrying out the necessary repair. Assessment during the postoperative period can detect pathological conditions such as thrombosis, regurgitation, and vegetations. In this chapter, normal appearance of some of the commonly implanted prosthetic valves in mitral and aortic position have been shown. In addition, pathological conditions such as prosthetic valve endocarditis leading to vegetations, thrombosis, and paravalvular leak have been depicted.

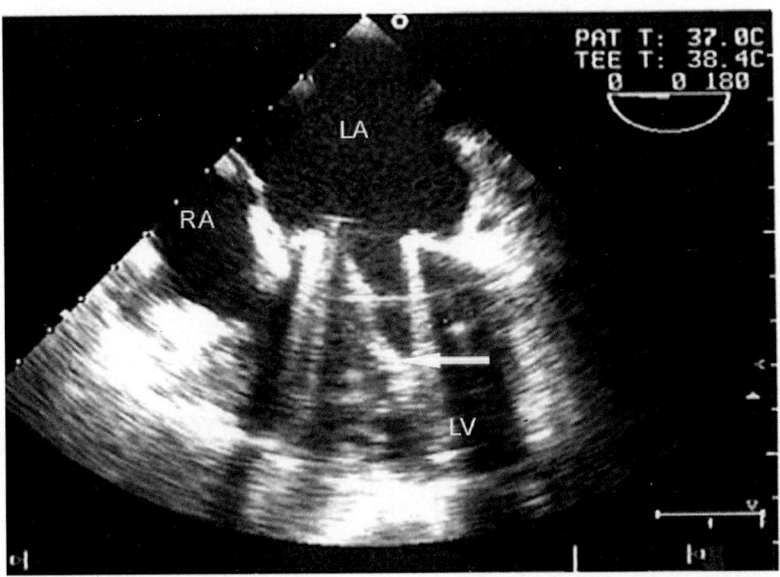

Figure 7.1. Appearance of the Bjork-Shiley tilting disc valve in the mitral position. Note the acoustic shadowing caused by the metallic disc (arrow). (LA: left atrium, RA: right atrium, LV: left ventricle)

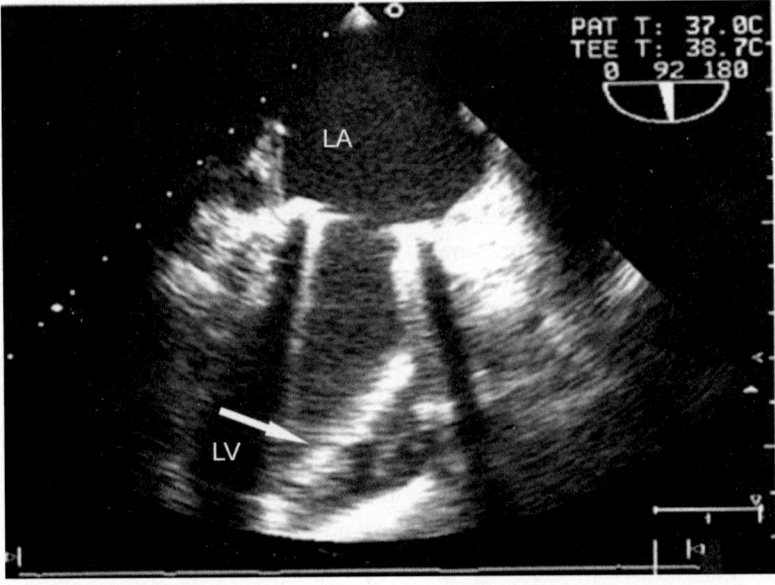

Figure 7.2. Acoustic shadowing (arrow) of the tilting disc deep in the left ventricle in a patient with Bjork-Shiley tilting disc valve in the mitral position.

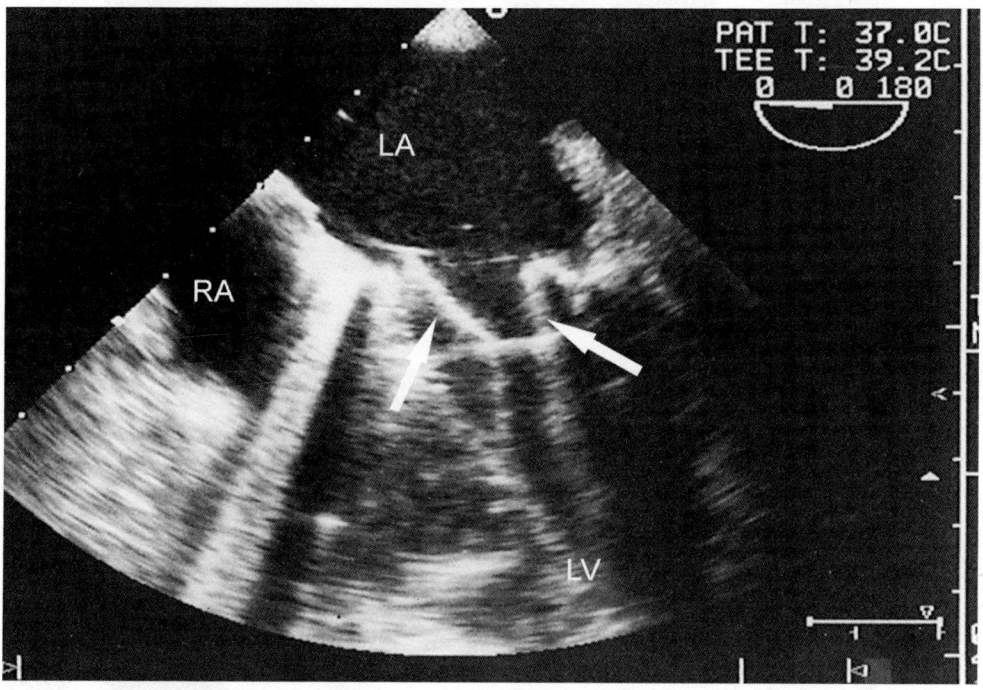

Figure 7.3. St. Jude prosthesis in the mitral position. Note the two discs (arrows). (LA: left atrium, RA: right atrium, LV: left ventricle)

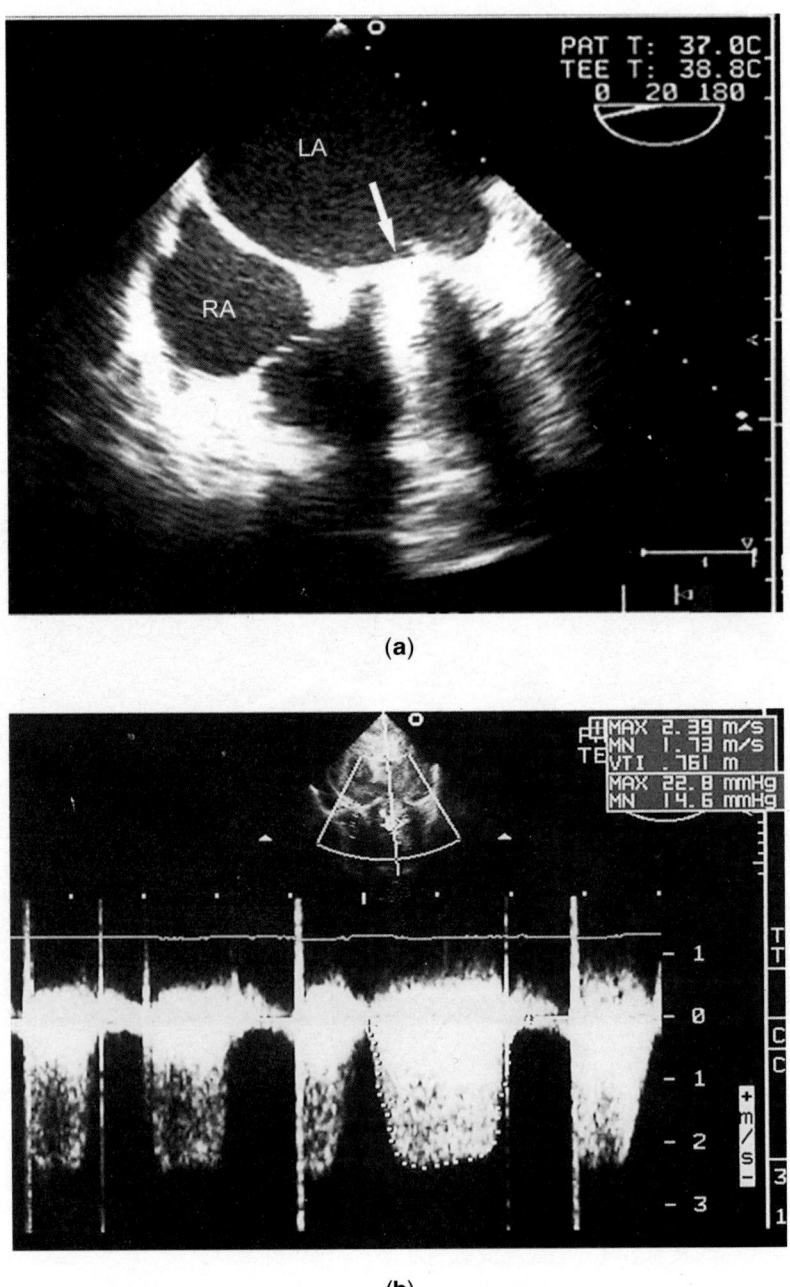

(a)

(b)

Figure 7.4 (a) Pannus formation (fibrous tissue overgrowth) on the St. Jude valve in the mitral position (arrow) causing prosthetic valve stenosis. **(b)** Note the continuous wave Doppler tracing across the mitral valve showing a large transmitral gradient and a prolonged pressure half time. (LA: left atrium, RA: right atrium)

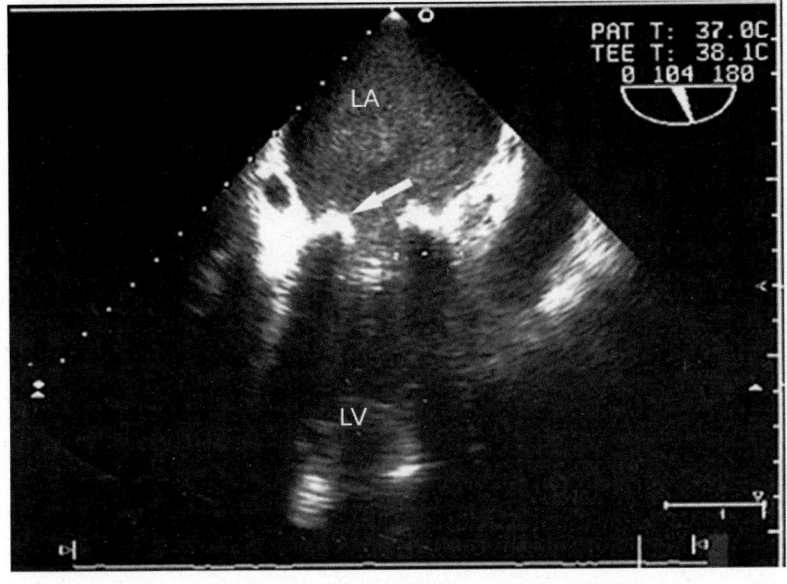

(a)

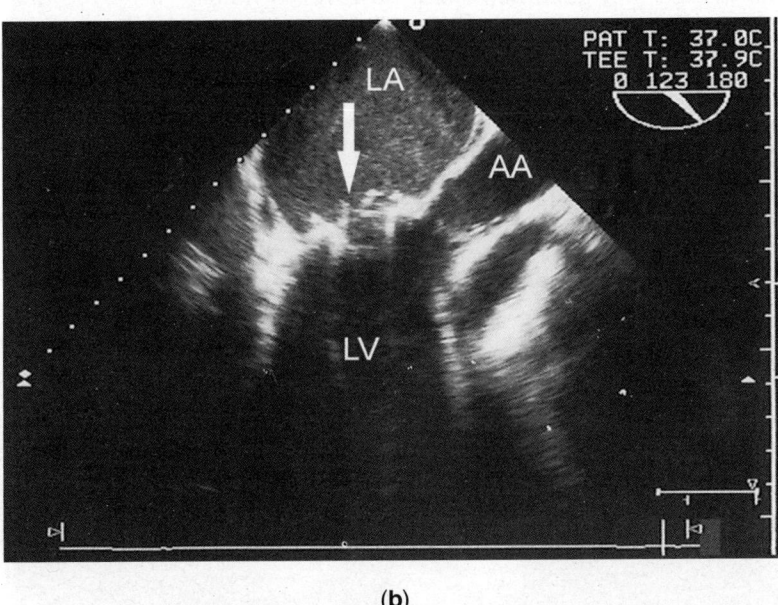

(b)

Figure 7.5 (a & b) Vegetations (arrows) in a patient with the Starr Edward Prosthesis in mitral position. Vegetations, suture material and fibrous strands growing from valves resemble each other and are differentiated based upon their location, appearance and movement. Vegetations have a characteristic off axis motion, which is independent and lags from the underlying tissue. (LA: left atrium, LV: left ventricle, AA: ascending aorta)

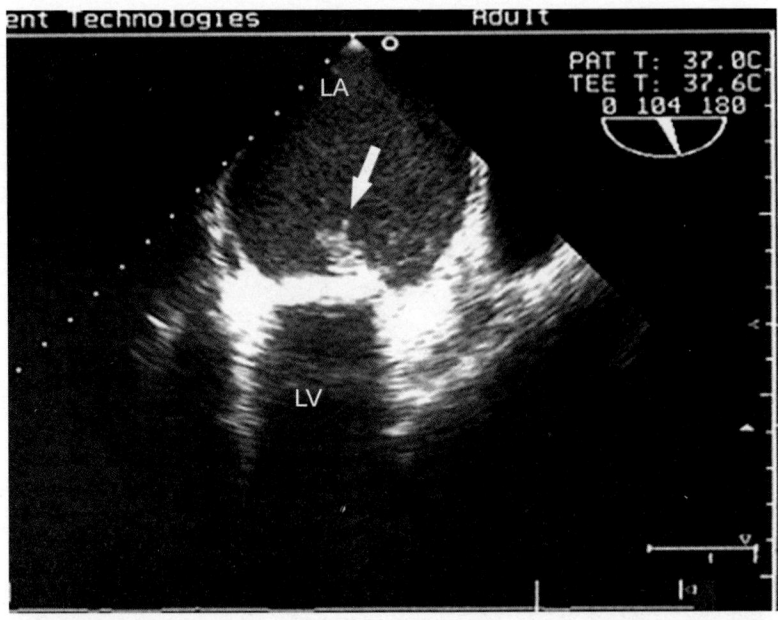

Figure 7.6. Prosthetic valve dysfunction due to formation of a large thrombus (arrow) in a patient with Bjork-Shiley tilting disc valve prosthesis in mitral position. A thrombus is usually large in size and generally fixed, however, if mobile, it moves along with the underlying structure to which it is attached. (LA: left atrium, LV: left ventricle)

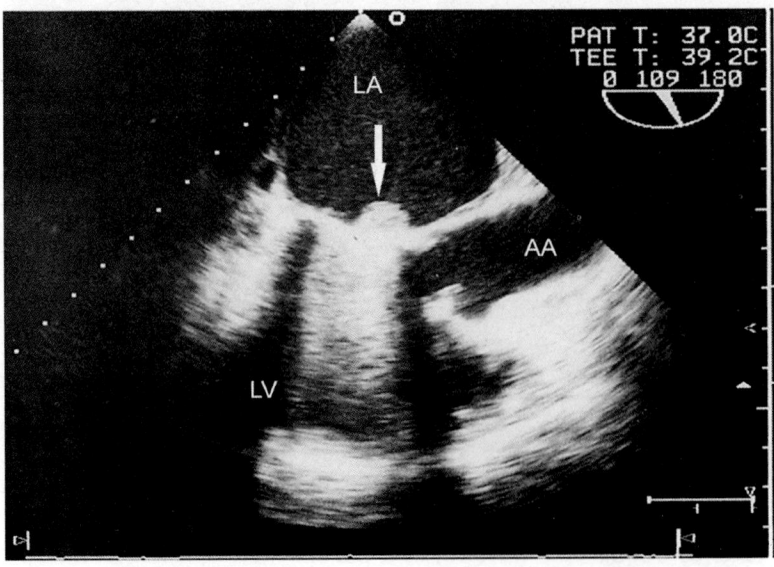

Figure 7.7. Prosthetic valve thrombosis (arrow) in a patient with the St.Jude's prosthesis in mitral position. (LA: left atrium, LV: left ventricle, AA: ascending aorta)

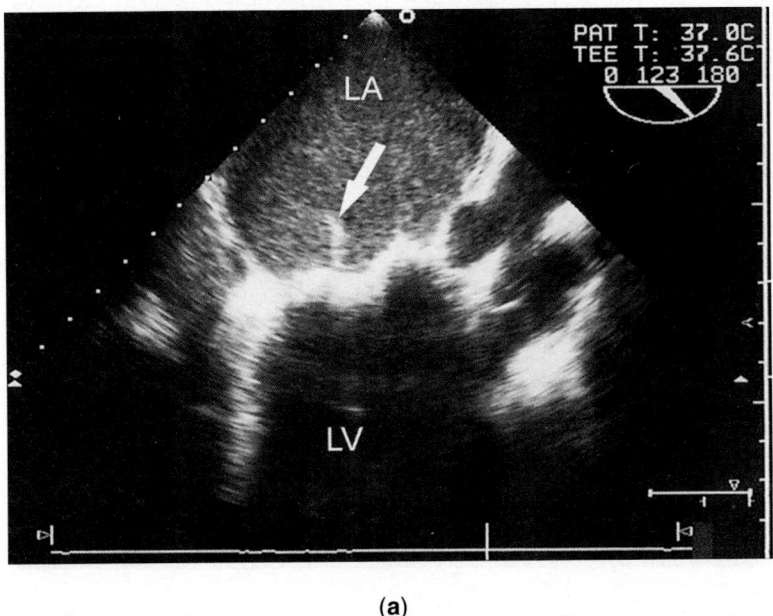

(a)

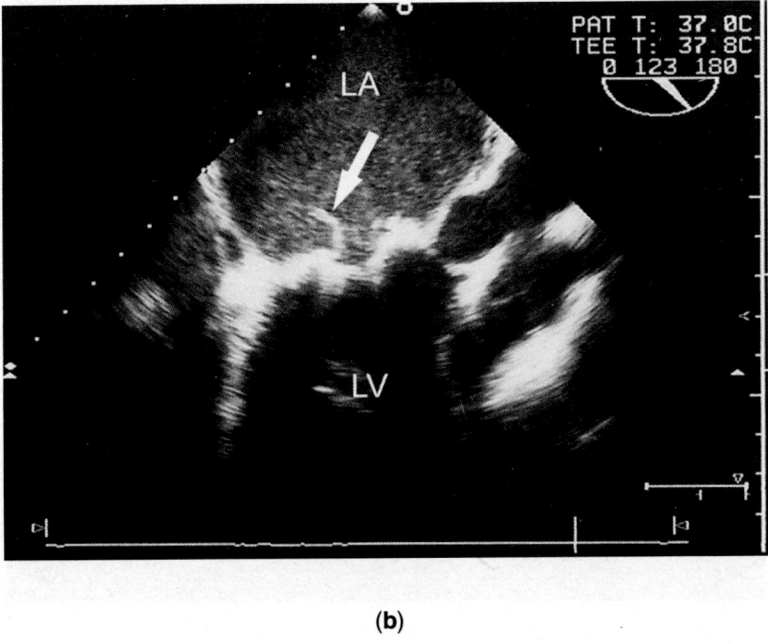

(b)

Figure 7.8 (a & b) Mobile vegetations (arrow) over tilting disc prothesis in mitral position.

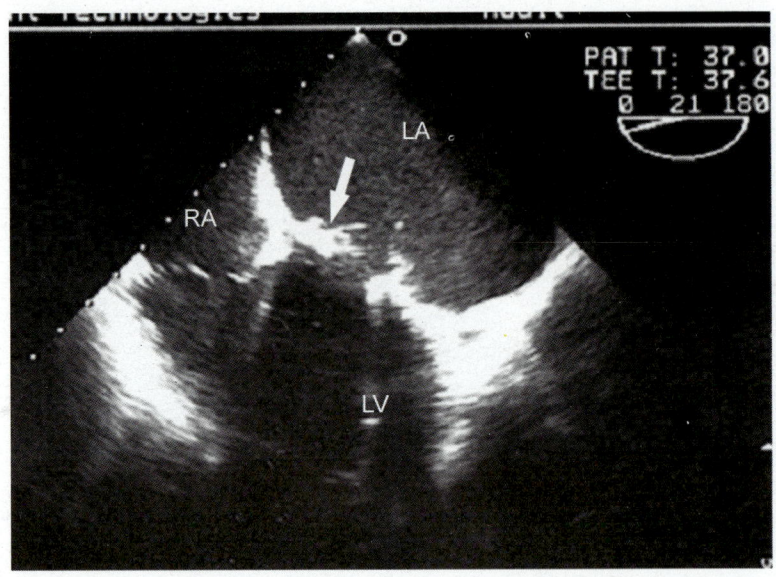

Figure 7.9. Formation of large vegetations (arrow) in a patient with a tilting disc prosthesis in the mitral position. (LA: left atrium, RA: right atrium, LV: left ventricle)

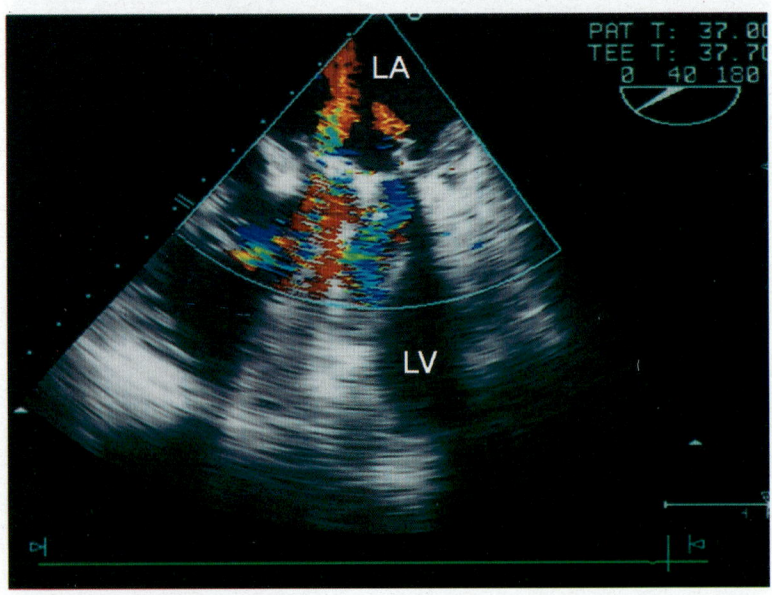

Figure 7.10. Prosthetic valve thrombosis causing mitral regurgitation. (LA: left atrium, LV left ventricle)

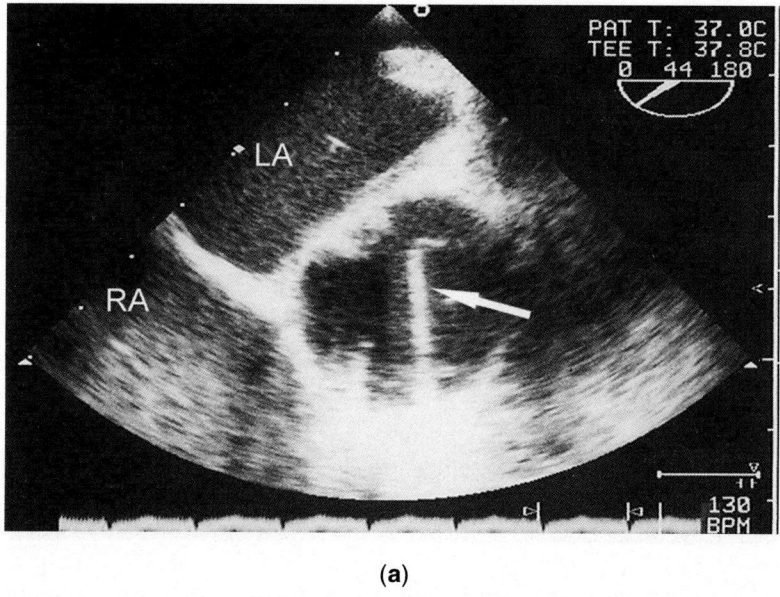

(a)

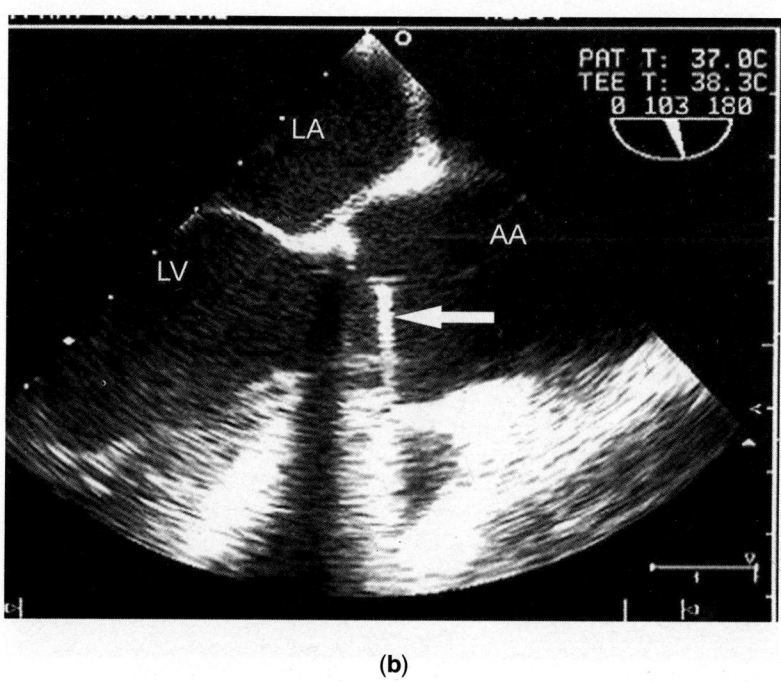

(b)

Figure 7.11 Bjork-Shiley tilting disc valve in the aortic position. Note the appearance of disc (arrow) in short **(a)** and long **(b)** axes. (LA: left atrium, RA: right atrium, LV: left ventricle, AA: ascending aorta)

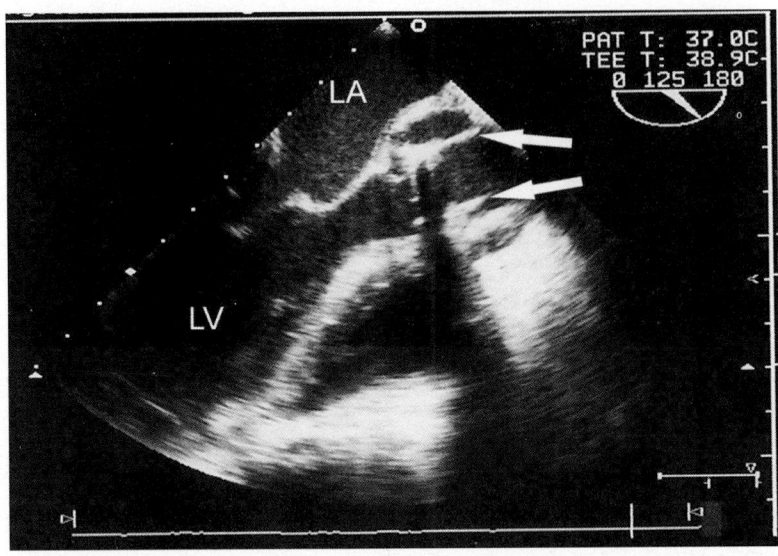

Figure 7.12. A patient with St. Jude bi-leaflet prosthesis in the aortic position. Note the two leaflets (arrows). (LA: left atrium, LV: left ventricle)

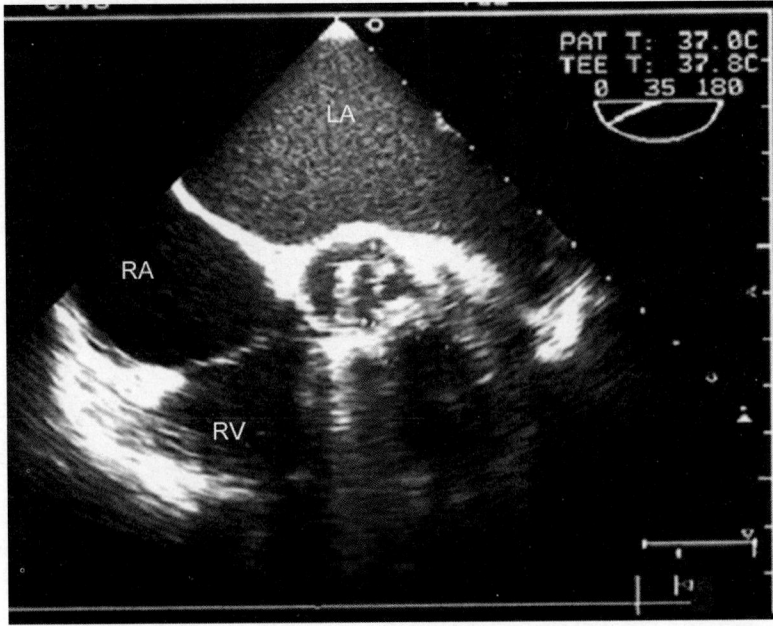

Figure 7.13. Appearance of the St. Jude bi-leaflet aortic prosthesis in short axis view showing the two leaflets. (LA: left atrium, RA: right atrium, RV: right ventricle)

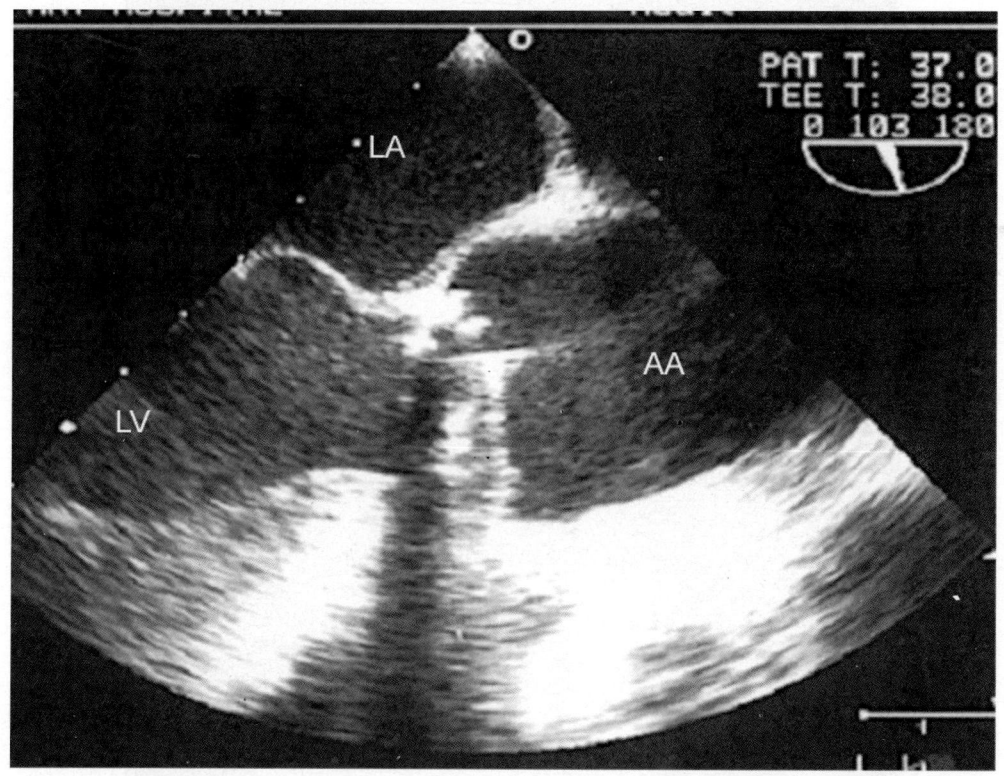

Figure 7.14. Vegetations over a tilting disc aortic valve prosthesis. (LA: left atrium, LV: left ventricle, AA: ascending aorta)

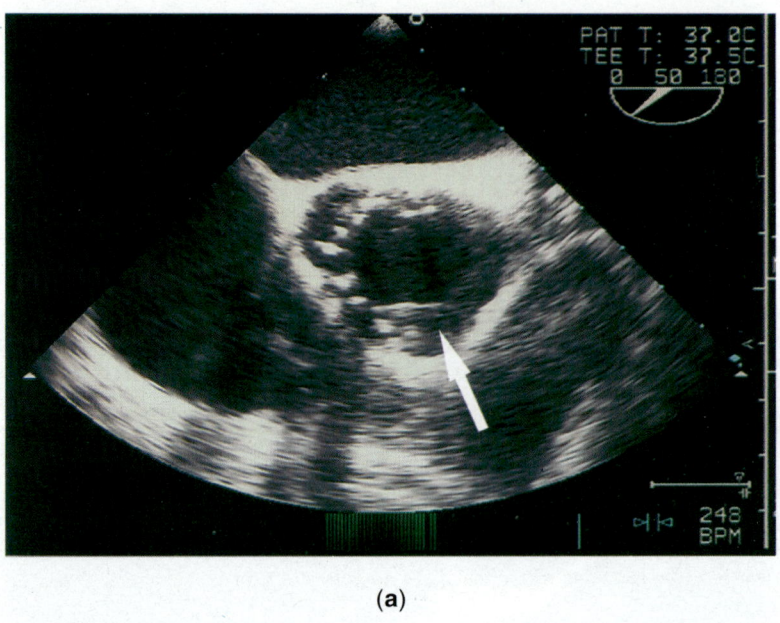

(a)

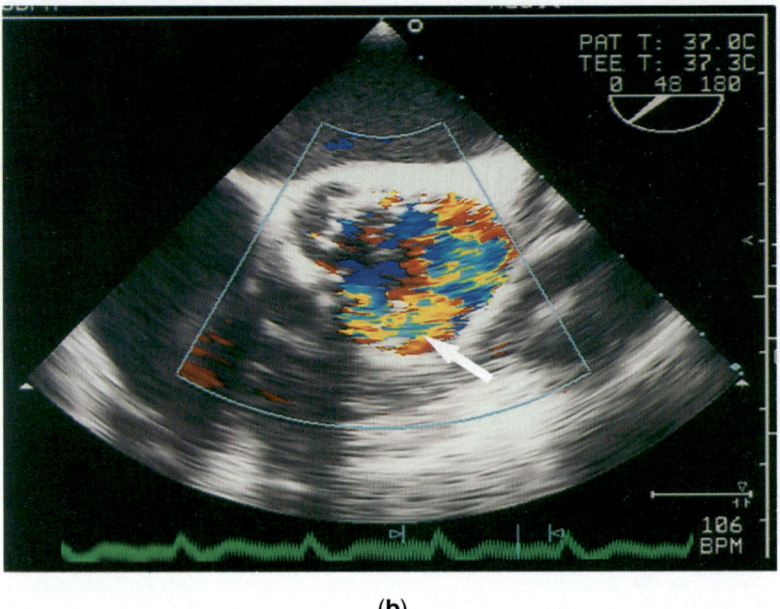

(b)

Figure 7.15. Paraprosthetic aortic regurgitation in a patient with aortic homograft. Note the paravalvular space (arrow) **(a)** and the regurgitant jet through that area (arrow) **(b)**.

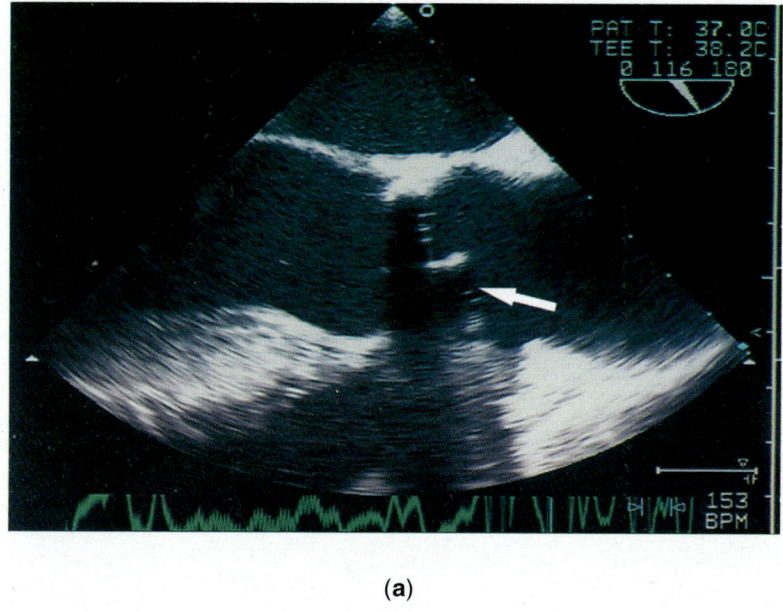

(a)

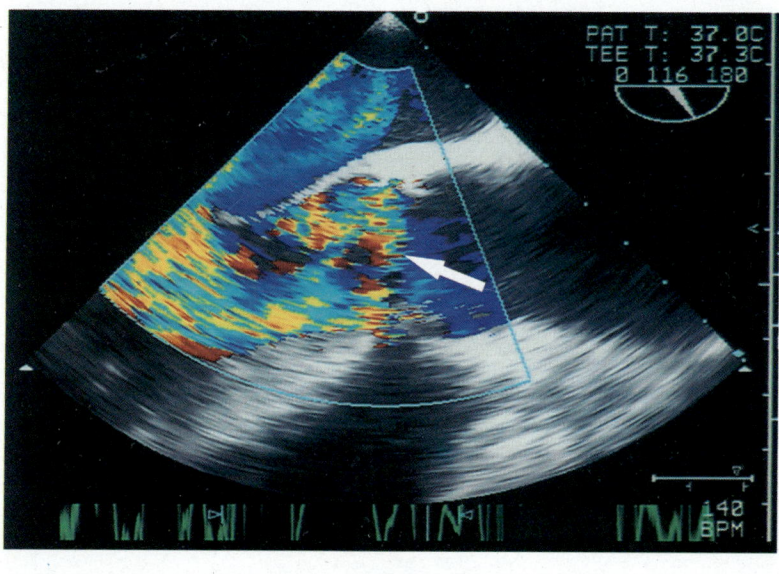

(b)

Figure 7.16. Appearance of the paraprosthetic space (arrow) **(a)** and aortic regurgitation (arrow) **(b)** in long axis view.

Chapter 8

ASSESSMENT OF CARDIAC VEGETATIONS

The diagnostic echocardiographic feature of infective endocarditis is presence of vegetation. A cardiac vegetation is a small mass consisting of fibrin, blood cells and microorganisms. Vegetations appear as mobile echo-dense masses that show wide variation in size and shape from a few millimeters to several centimeters in length. A vegetation may be confused with a thrombus and can be differentiated on the basis of its mobility that has a free floating characteristic. Thrombus on the other hand is generally fixed and if it moves, movement occurs along with the motion of the structure to which it is attached. Transoesophageal echocardiography (TOE) identifies smaller vegetations that can be missed on transthoracic echocardiography. Valve leaflets can be damaged which commonly leads to valve regurgitation. Extension of infection to the perivalvular area can result in the formation of an abscess or aneurysm. TOE examination should include careful assessment with short and long axis views. Colour Doppler is used to detect regurgitation. In this chapter, images showing possible vegetations on the mitral and aortic valves have been included.

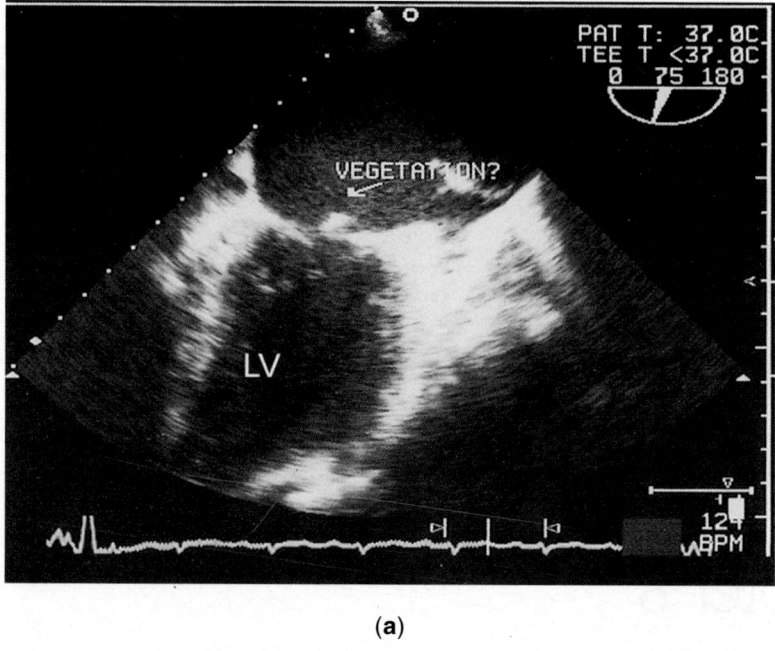

(a)

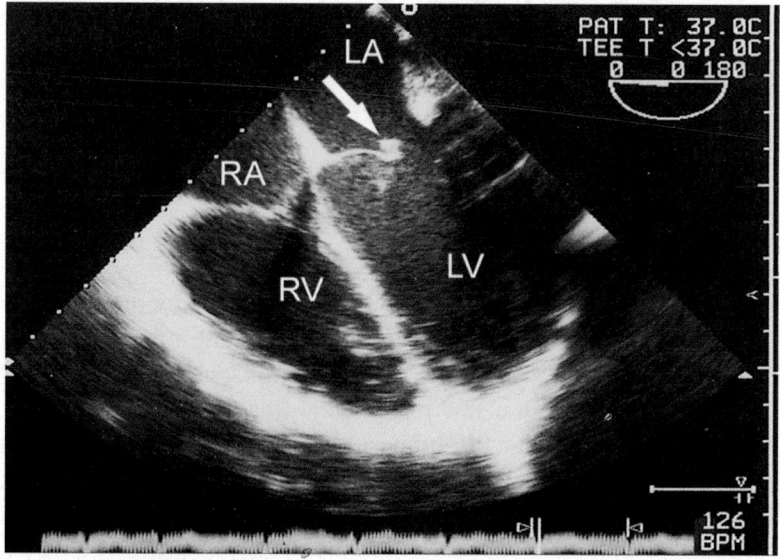

(b)

Figure 8.1. A patient with native valve endocarditis. Note the vegetation (arrow) on the mitral leaflet. **(a)** two chamber view, **(b)** four chamber view.

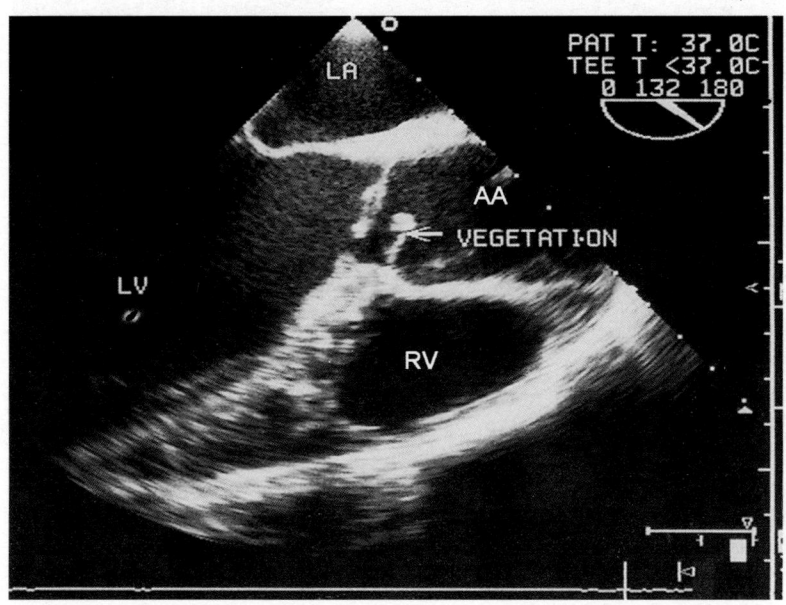

Figure 8.2. Multiple vegetations over the aortic valve in a patient with native aortic valve endocarditis. (LA: left atrium, LV: left ventricle, RV: right ventricle, AA: ascending aorta)

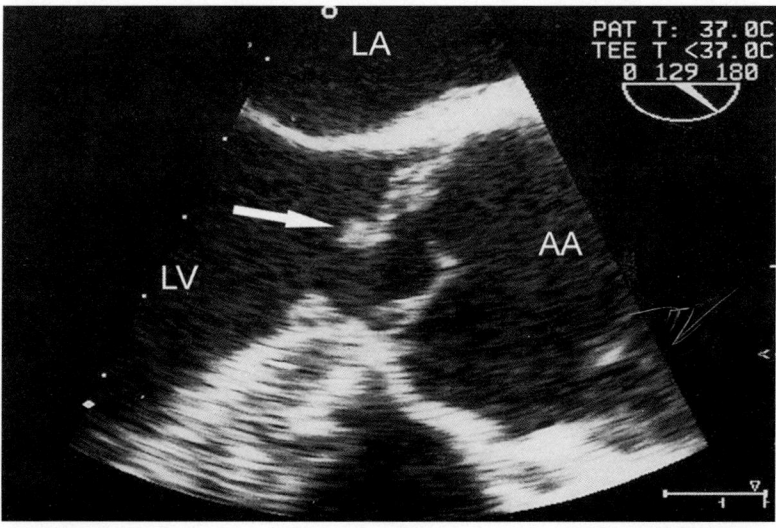

Figure 8.3. Longitudinal view of the aortic valve showing vegetations (arrow) over the aortic leaflets. Note the abnormal appearance of the incompetent aortic leaflets. (LA: left atrium, LV: left ventricle, AA: ascending aorta)

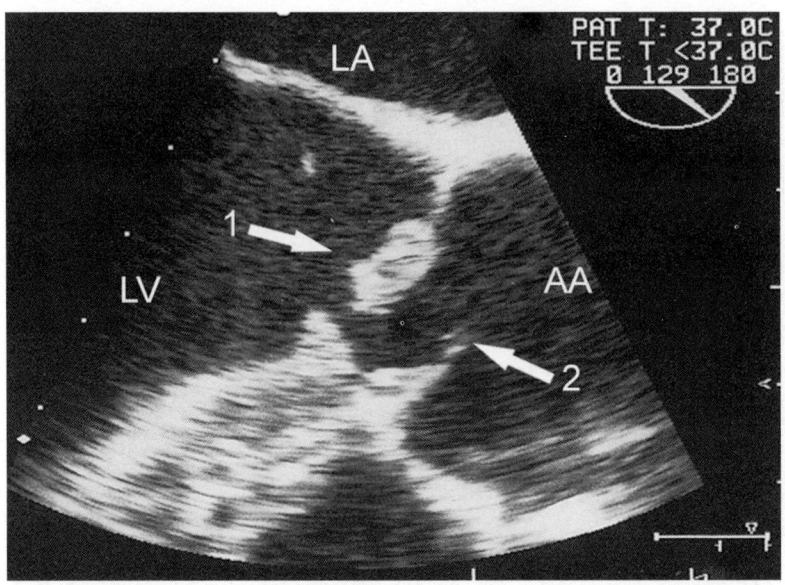

Figure 8.4. Longitudinal view of the aortic valve showing vegetations (arrow 1) over the aortic valve in a patient with aortic valve endocarditis. Note the complete destruction of the other aortic leaflet (arrow 2). (LA: left atrium, LV: left ventricle, AA: ascending aorta)

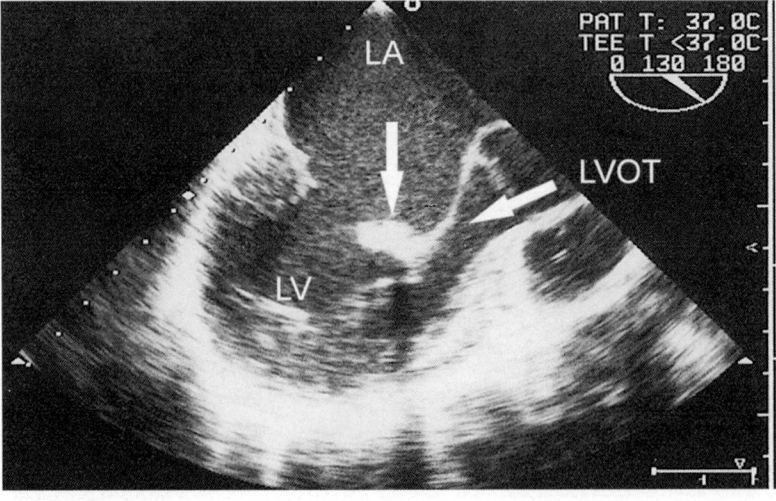

Figure 8.5. Longitudinal view of the left heart showing a large vegetation (arrow) over the anterior mitral leaflet. (LA: left atrium, LV: left ventricle, LVOT: left ventricular outflow tract)

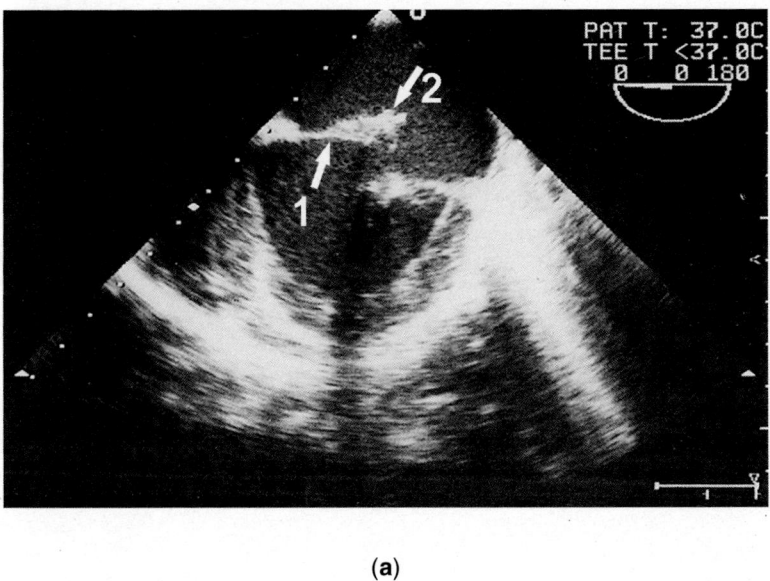

(a)

(b)

Figure 8.6 (a & b) Prolapse of the anterior mitral leaflet (arrow 1) in a patient with large vegetation over the anterior mitral leaflet (arrow 2).

Chapter 9

EVALUATION OF CONGENITAL HEART DISEASE

In adults with congenital heart disease the transthoracic approach is occasionally limited by chest deformities, obesity or pulmonary disease. In such circumstances trans-oesophageal echocardiography (TOE) is helpful as it provides a better ecocardiographic window.

During surgery, TOE is useful for confirming adequacy of the repair, detection and quantification of the intracardiac residual shunts and gradients. Such information helps making decisions for modifying the method of surgical repair. TOE also assists in adequate cardiac de-airing before the aorta is unclamped. TOE is useful for guiding transcatheter closure of the atrial and ventricular septal defects. It helps to define the margin and size of the defect and in assisting device deployment. TOE is thus an extremely important tool in the perioperative management of congenital heart disease.

This chapter illustrates trans-oesophageal appearance of some commonly encountered congenital heart defects.

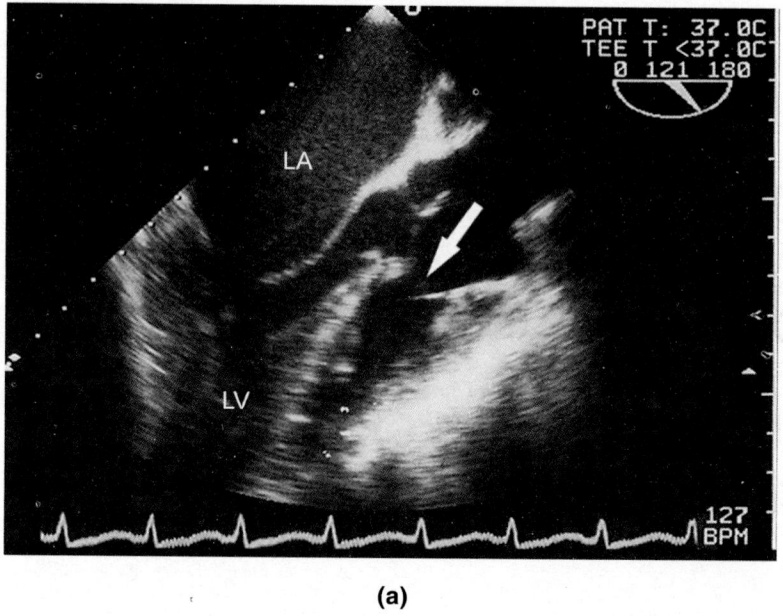

(a)

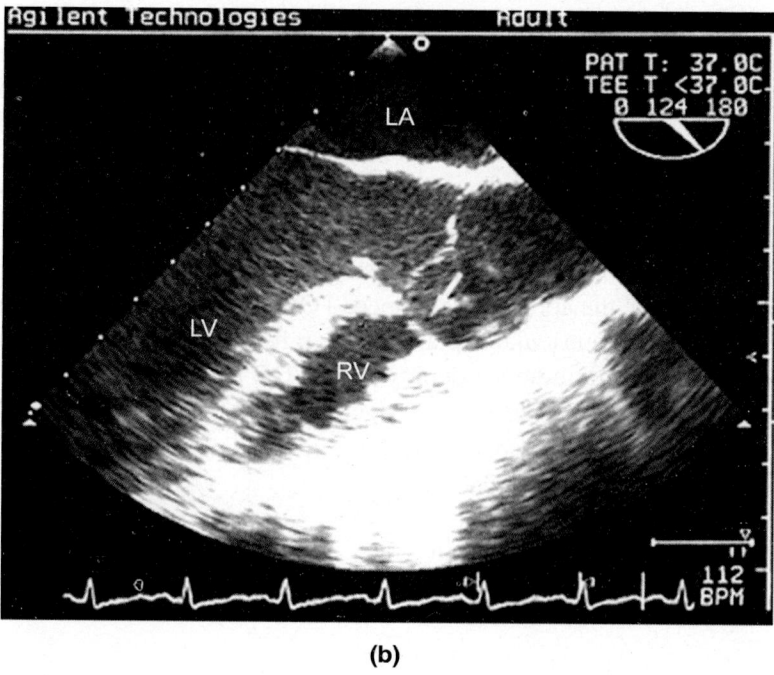

(b)

Figure 9.1 (a & b) Longitudinal view of the left heart and proximal aorta showing outlet ventricular septal defect. Note the prolapsing aortic sinus (arrows). (LA: left atrium, LV: left ventricle, RV: right ventricle)

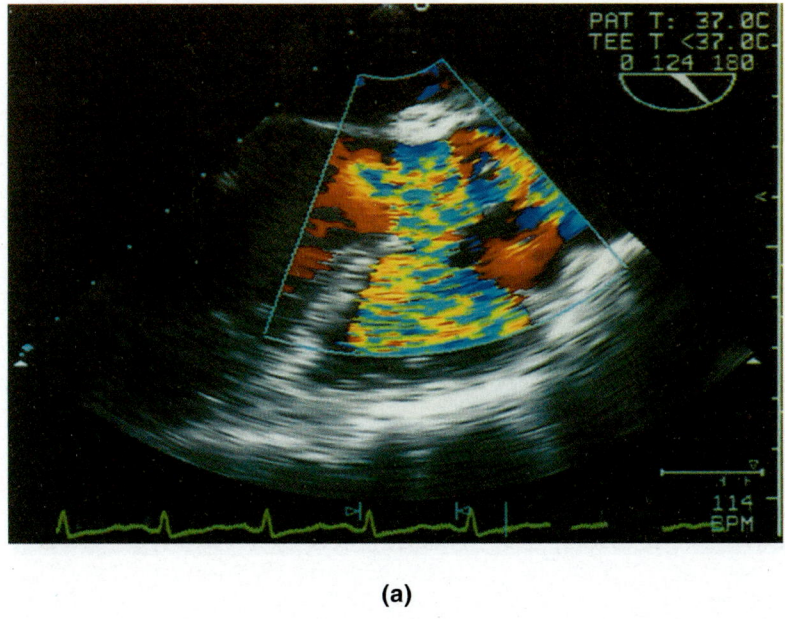

(a)

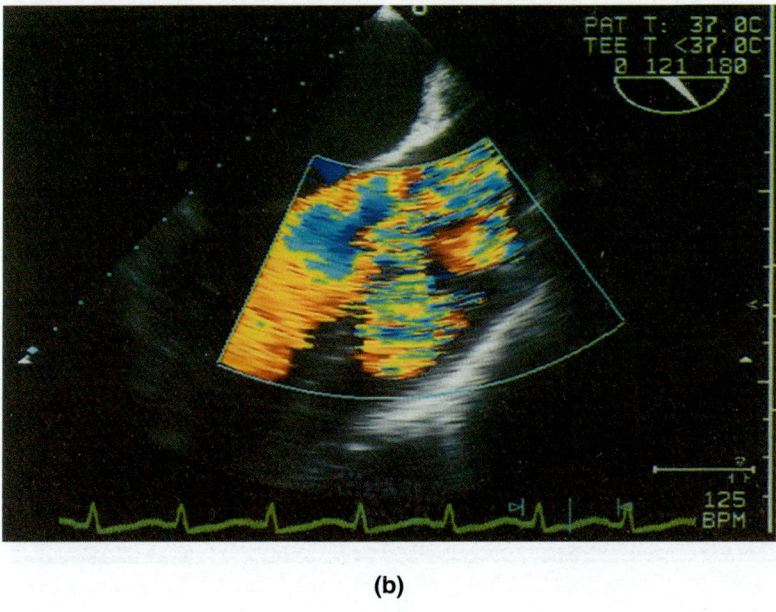

(b)

Figure 9.2 (a & b) Systolic colour flow across the outlet ventricular septal defect shown in Fig 9.1 revealing a large left to right shunt across the defect.

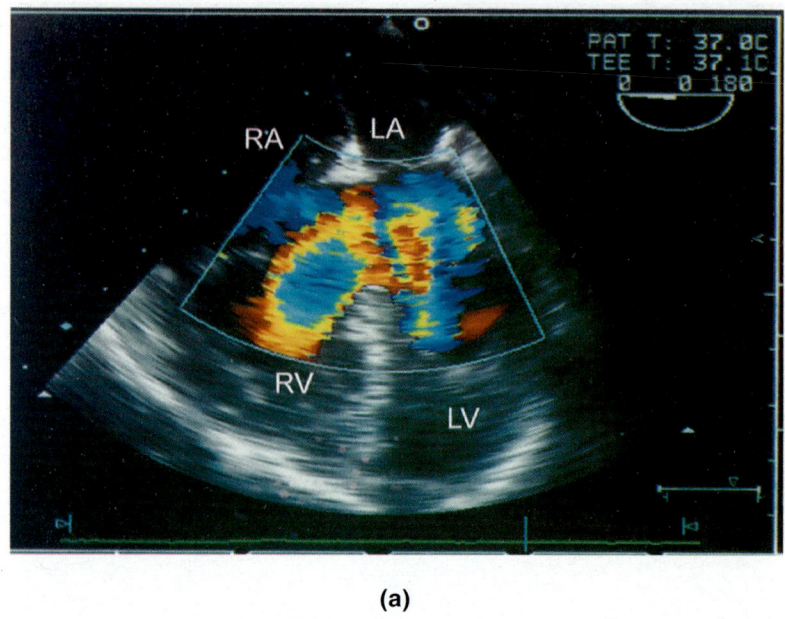

(a)

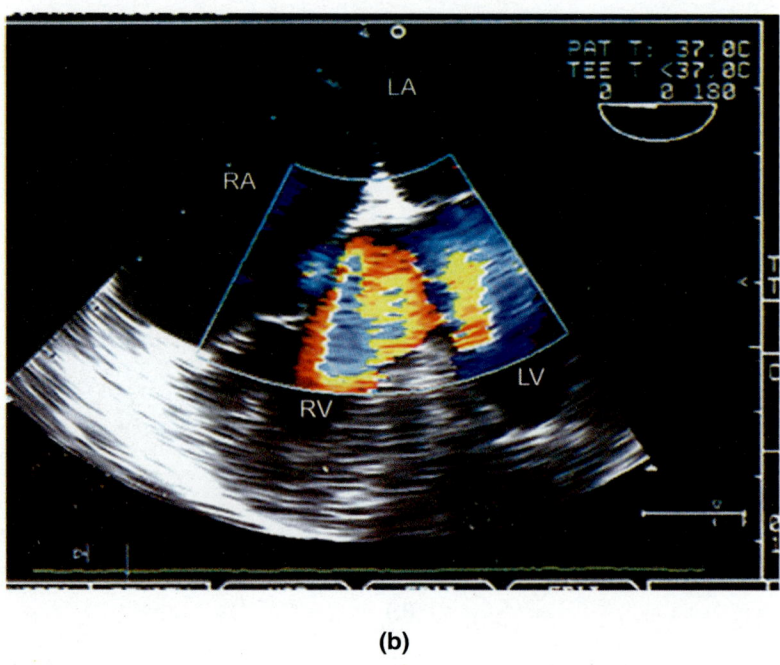

(b)

Figure 9.3. Midoesophageal four chamber view showing the colour flow across the muscular ventricular septal defect. Note the left to right ventricular shunt. (LA: left atrium, LV: left ventricle, RA: right atrium, RV: right ventricle)

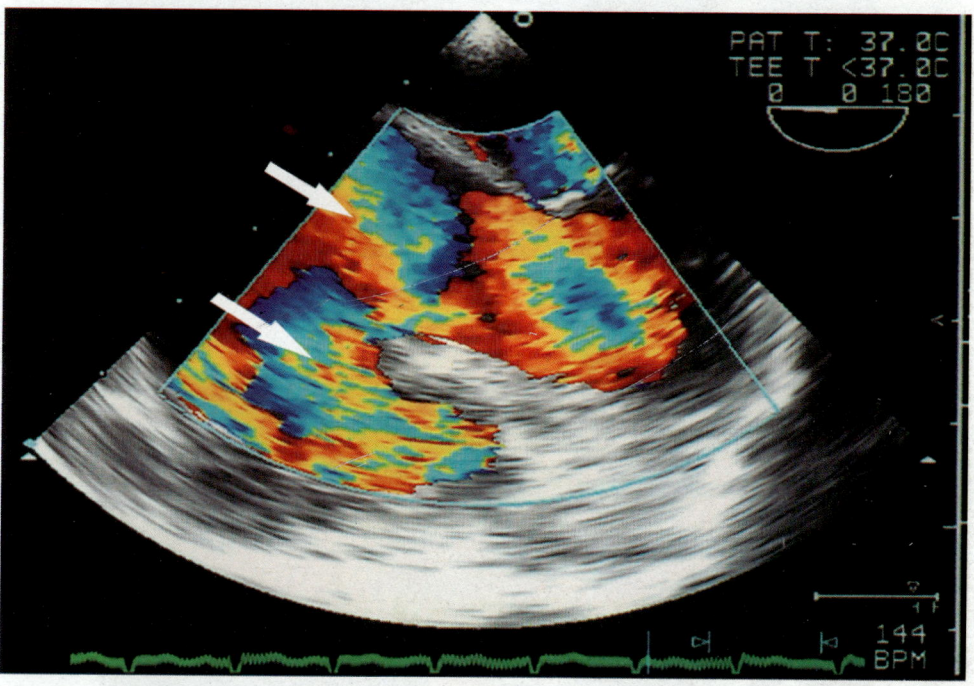

Figure 9.4. Midoesophageal four chamber view showing the perimembranous ventricular septal defect. Colour flow across the defect shows two jets (arrows); an upper left ventricular to right atrial shunt and a lower left to right ventricular shunt.

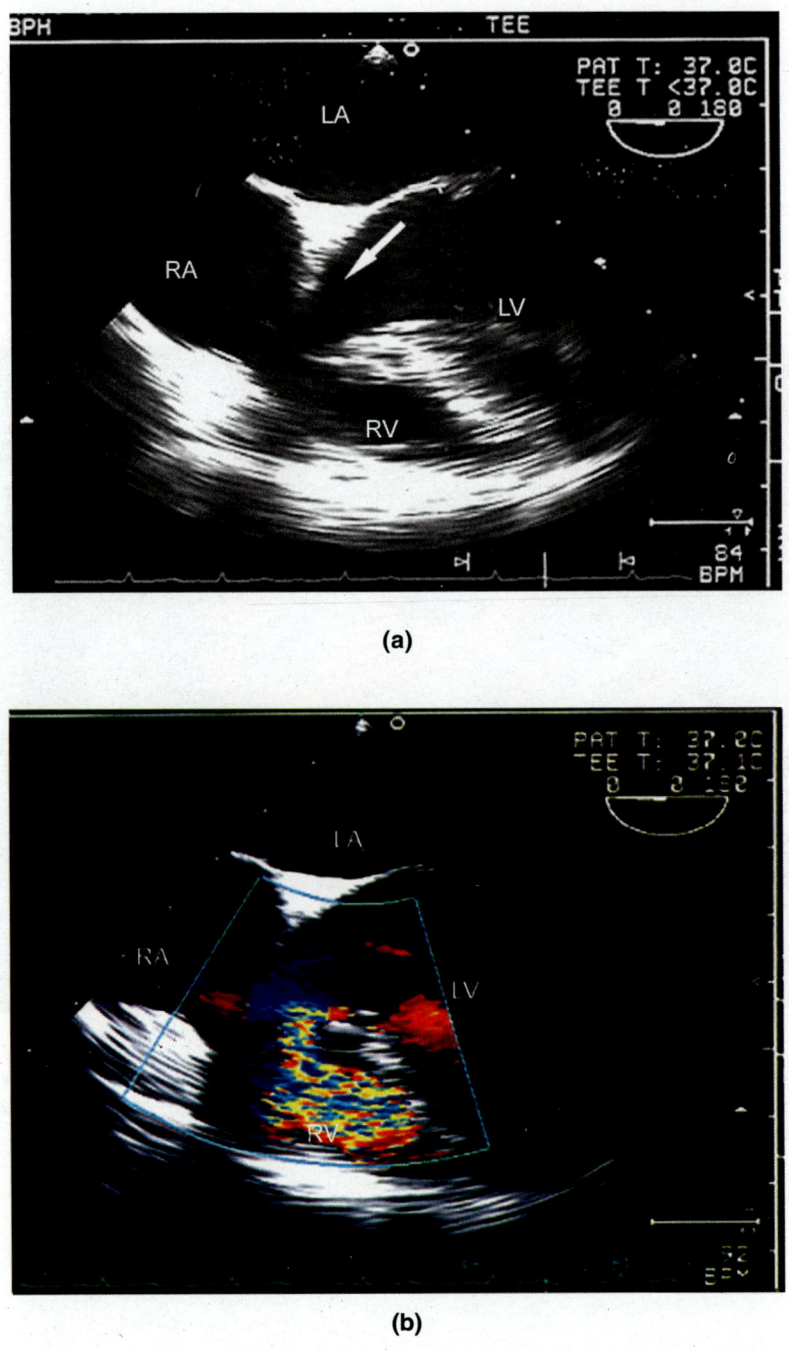

(a)

(b)

Figure 9.5. Inlet ventricular septal defect **(a)** with aneurysm formation (arrow) and the colour flow across it **(b)**. (LA: left atrium, RA: right atrium, LV: left ventricle, RV: right ventricle)

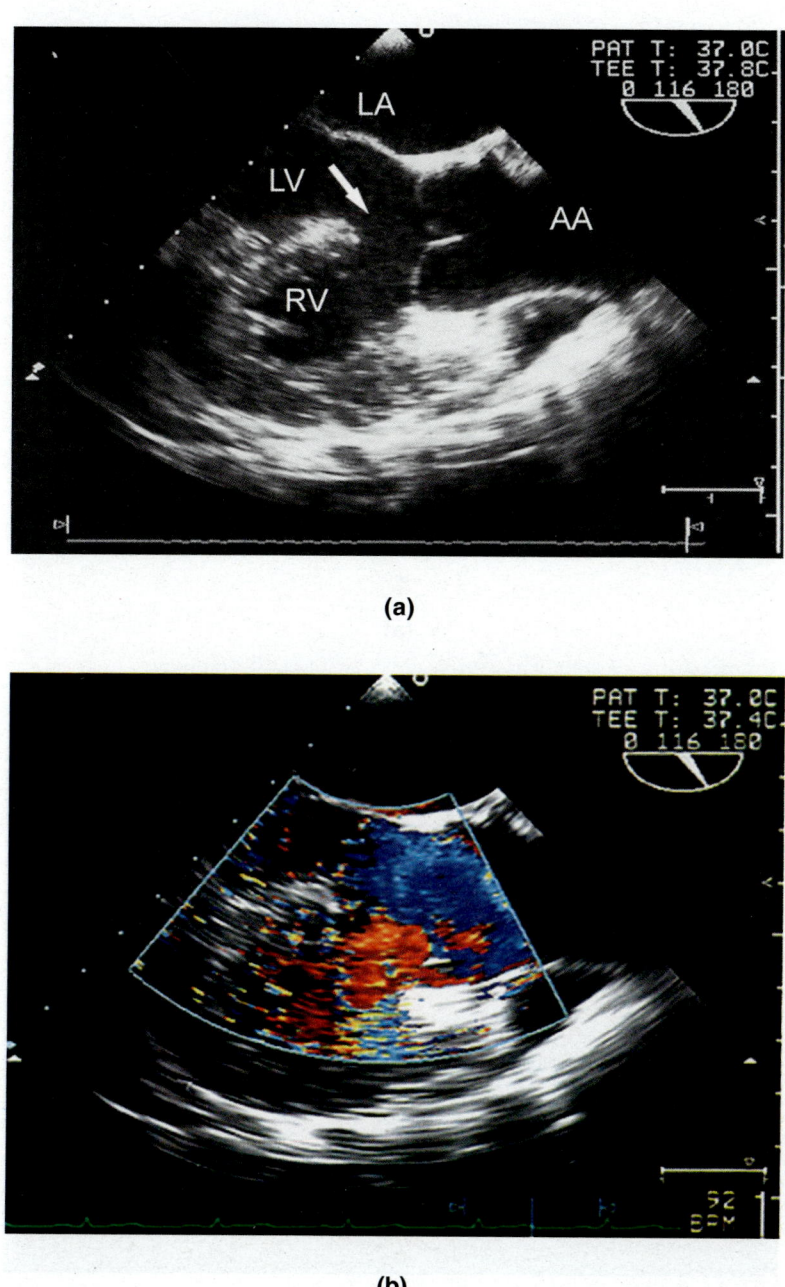

(a)

(b)

Figure 9.6 (a) Longitudinal view of the left heart and the proximal aorta showing a large sub-aortic ventricular septal defect (arrow) in a patient with tetralogy of Fallot with 50% aortic over-ride. **(b)** Colour flow across the defect and over-riding aorta shows streaming of blood from both right and left ventricles into the aorta. (LA: left atrium, LV: left ventricle, RV: right ventricle, AA: ascending aorta)

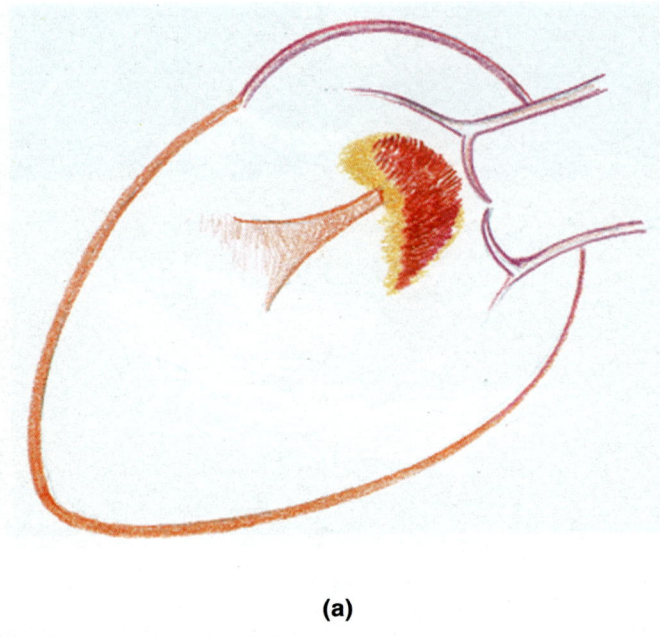

(a)

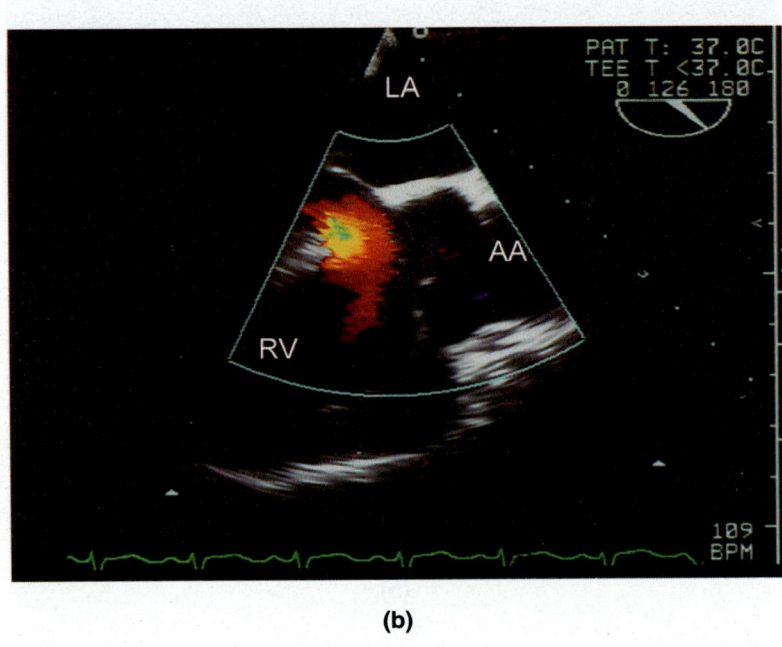

(b)

Figure 9.7 (a & b) Ventricular septal defect caused by mal-alignment of the aorta. Note the absence of turbulence due to a relatively large defect size causing equalisation of the pressure in both the chambers and a low velocity left to right shunt across the defect. **(a)** Shows artist's impression. (LA: left atrium, RV: right ventricle, AA: ascending aorta)

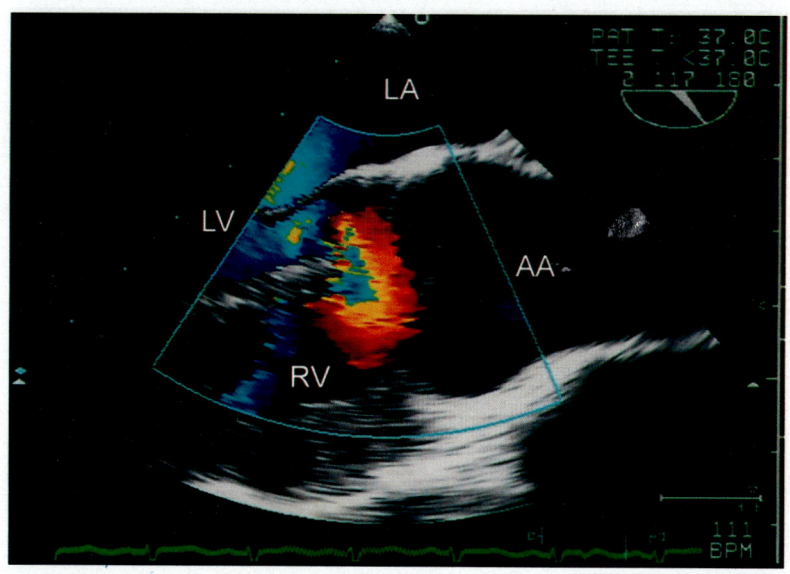

Figure 9.8. Aortic over-ride and malaligned ventricular septal defect in a patient with tetralogy of Fallot. (LA: left atrium, LV: left ventricle, RV: right ventricle, AA: ascending aorta)

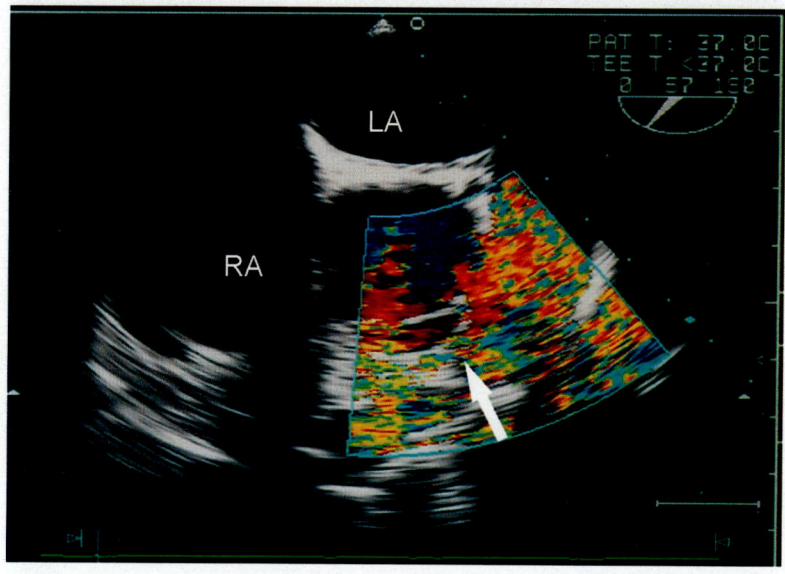

Figure 9.9. Colour flow across the right ventricular outflow tract in a patient with tetralogy of Fallot showing turbulence (arrow) caused by the stenosed right ventricular infundibular area. (LA: Left atrium, RA: right atrium)

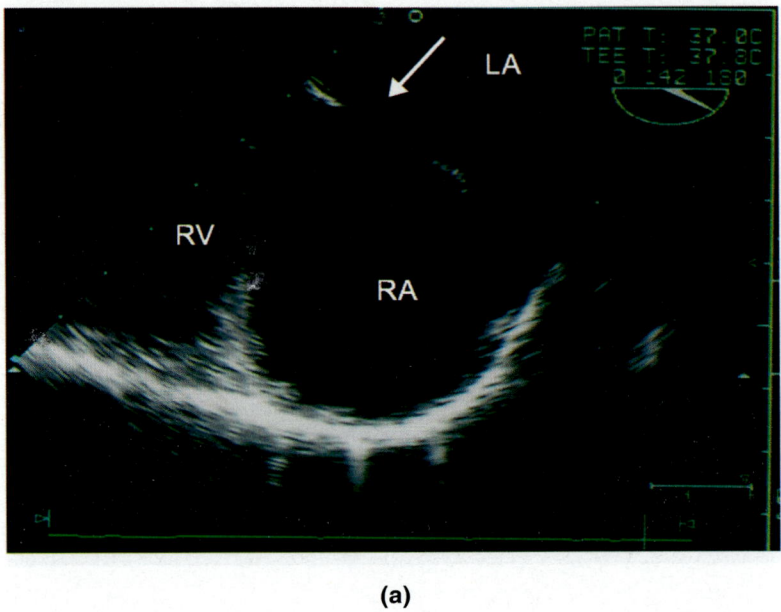

(a)

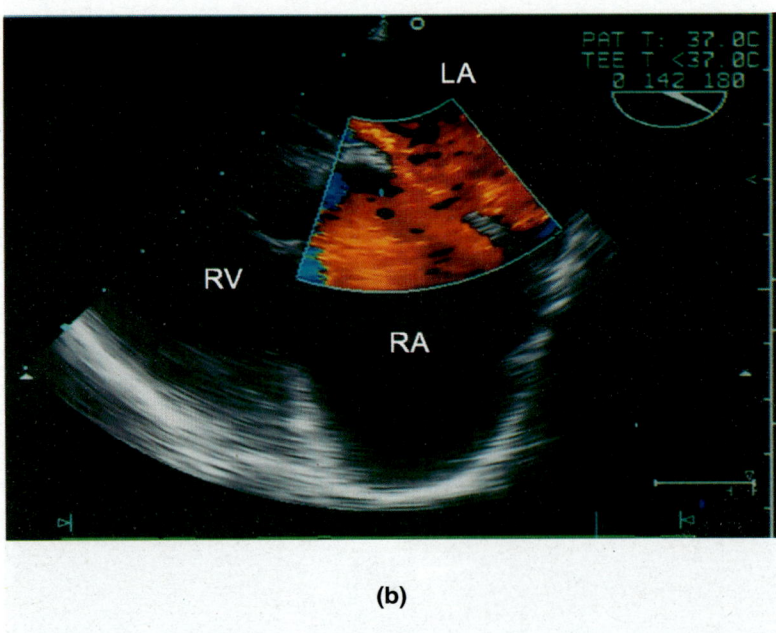

(b)

Figure 9.10. An ostium secundum atrial septal defect (arrow). Note the margins of the defect **(a)** and right to left atrial shunt on colour flow **(b)** (RA: right atrium, LA: left atrium, RV: right ventricle)

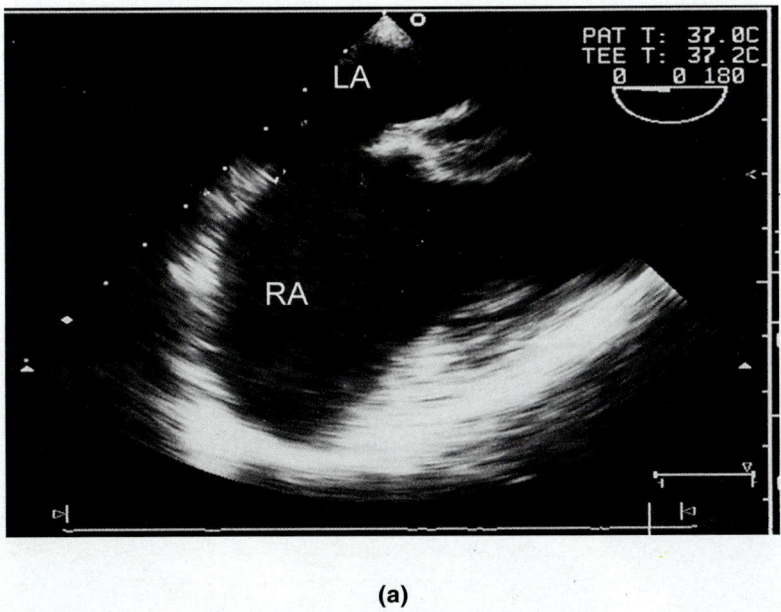

(a)

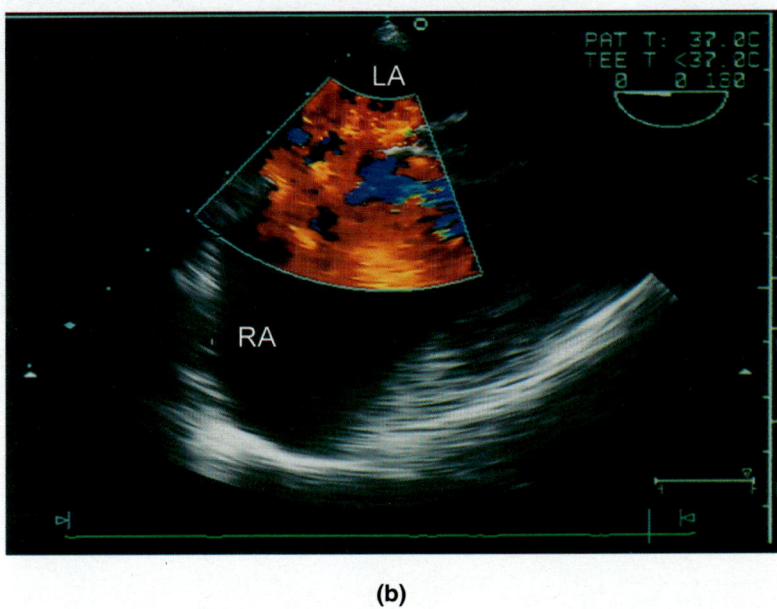

(b)

Figure 9.11 (a) A large ostium secundum atrial septal defect. Note the margins of atrial septal defect which are relatively deficient. The patient had a bidirectional shunt due to significant pulmonary arterial hypertension (subsystemic). **(b)** shows the right to left component of the bidirectional flow in this patient. (RA: right atrium, LA: left atrium)

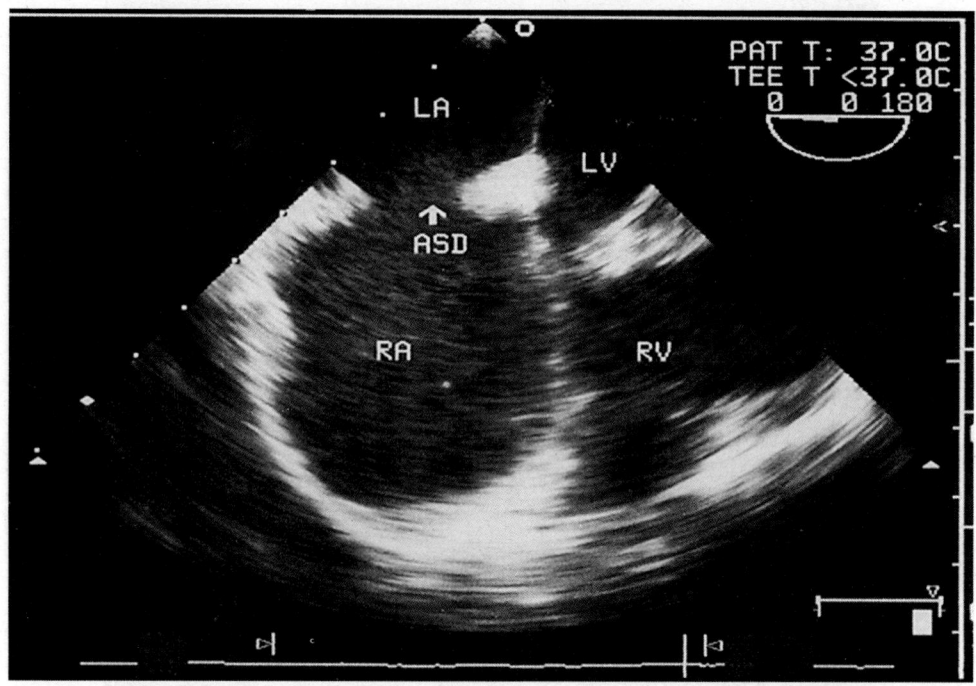

Figure 9.12. Modified four chamber view showing a large secundum atrial septal defect. (LA: left atrium, RA: right atrium, LV: left ventricle, RV: right ventricle, ASD: atrial septal defect.)

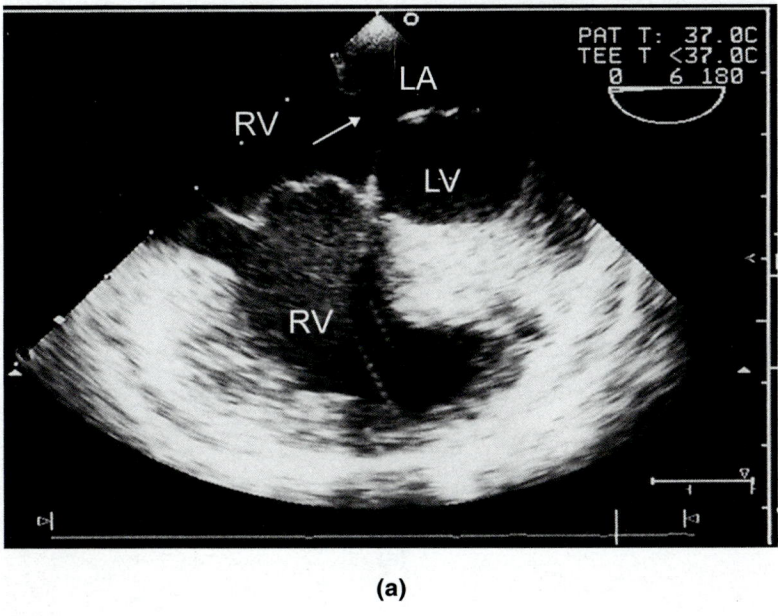

(a)

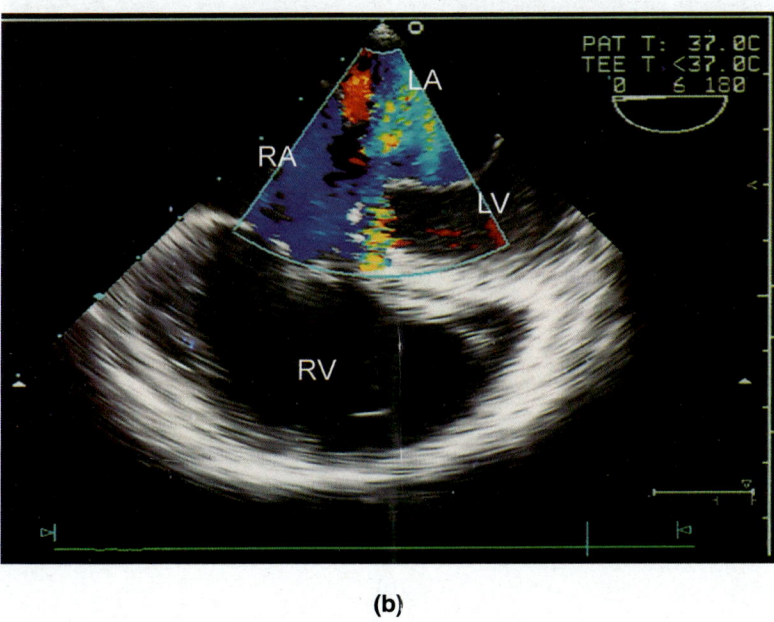

(b)

Figure 9.13 (a) Appearance of the ostium primum atrial septal defect (arrow). Note the volume overloaded right ventricle. **(b)** Colour flow across the defect shows a large left to right shunt across the defect. (LA: left atrium, RA: right atrium, LV: left ventricle, RV: right ventricle)

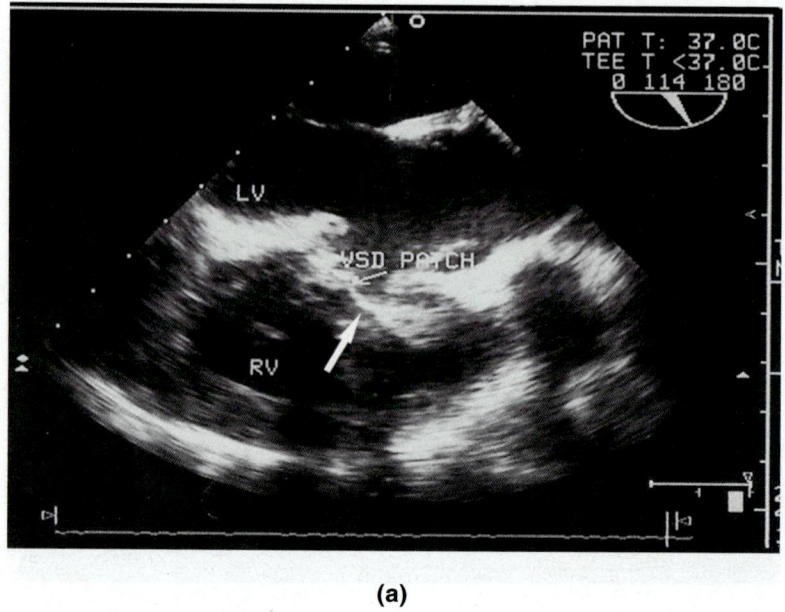

(a)

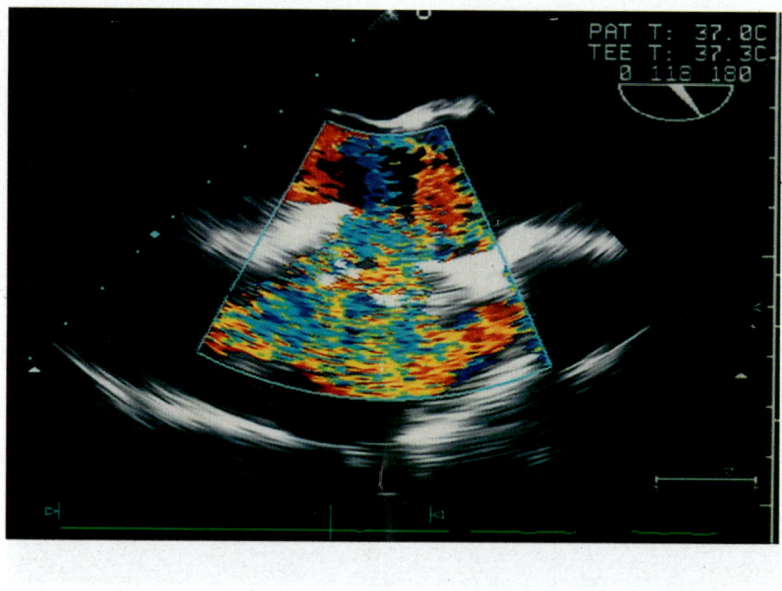

(b)

Figure 9.14. Images from a patient with tetrology of Fallot who underwent total intra-cardiac repair. Note the Dacron patch across the ventricular septal defect (arrow, **a**) Colour flow **(b)** shows a large residual shunt across the ventricular septal defect. (LA: left atrium, LV: left ventricle, RV: right ventricle)

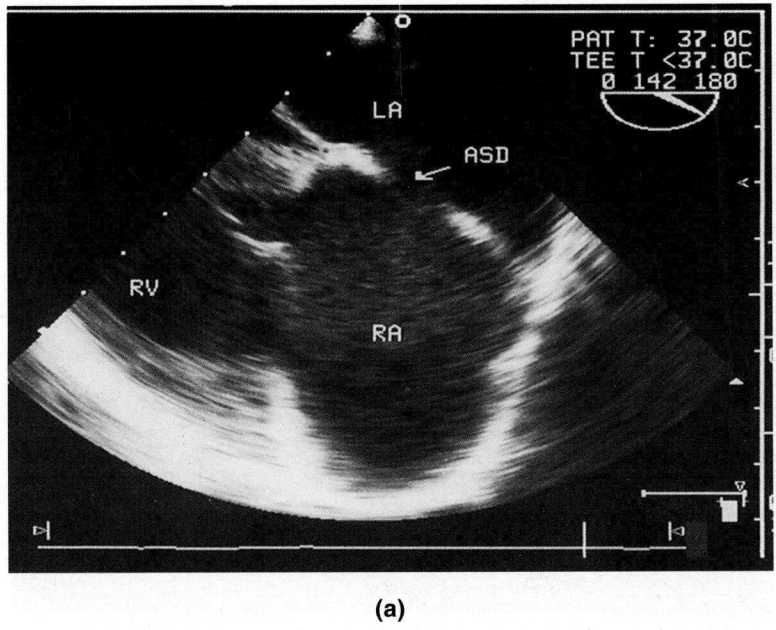

(a)

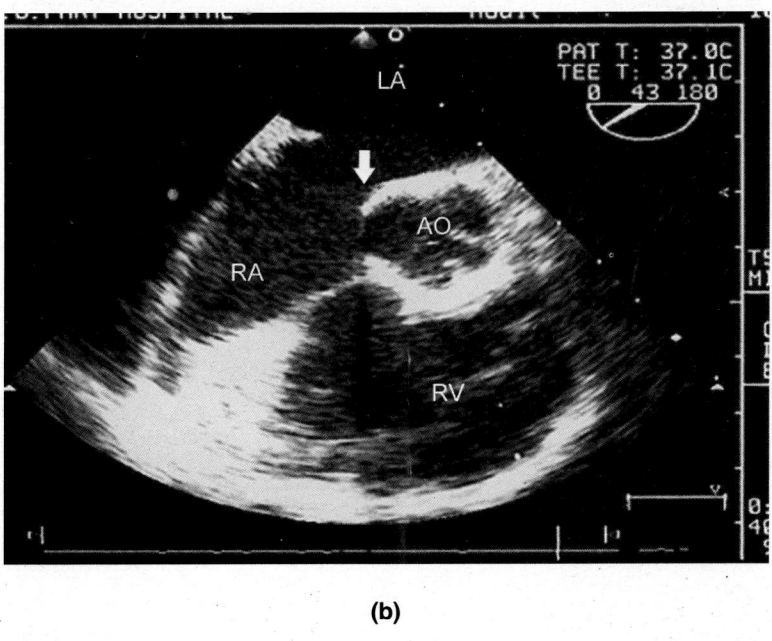

(b)

Figure 9.15. Appearance of the atrial septal defect in different views. Note the well formed superior and inferior margins **(a)** and deficient aortic margin (arrow, **b**) (LA: left atrium, RA: right atrium, AO: aorta, RV: right ventricle, ASD: atrial septal defect)

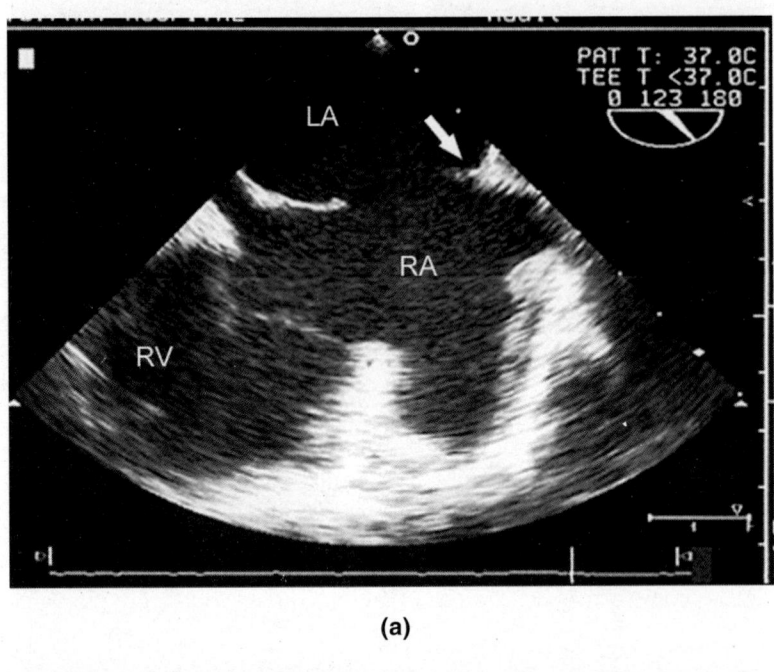

(a)

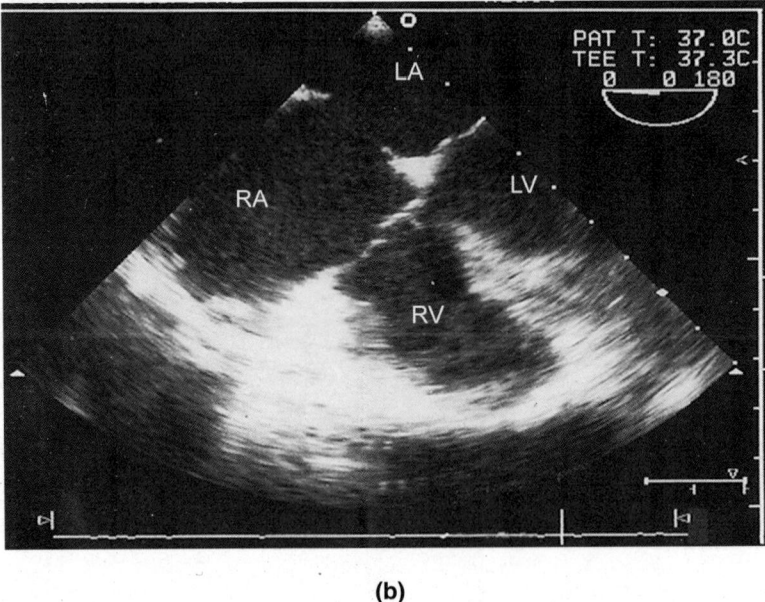

(b)

Figure 9.16. A large secundum atrial septal defect with inadequate superior margin in the bicaval view (arrow, **a**) although it appears adequate in the four chamber view **(b)**. Adequate margins is a pre-requisite for percutaneous device closure of atrial septal defect, and its absence necessitates surgical closure as in this case. (LA: left atrium, RA: right atrium, RV: right ventricle, LV: left ventricle)

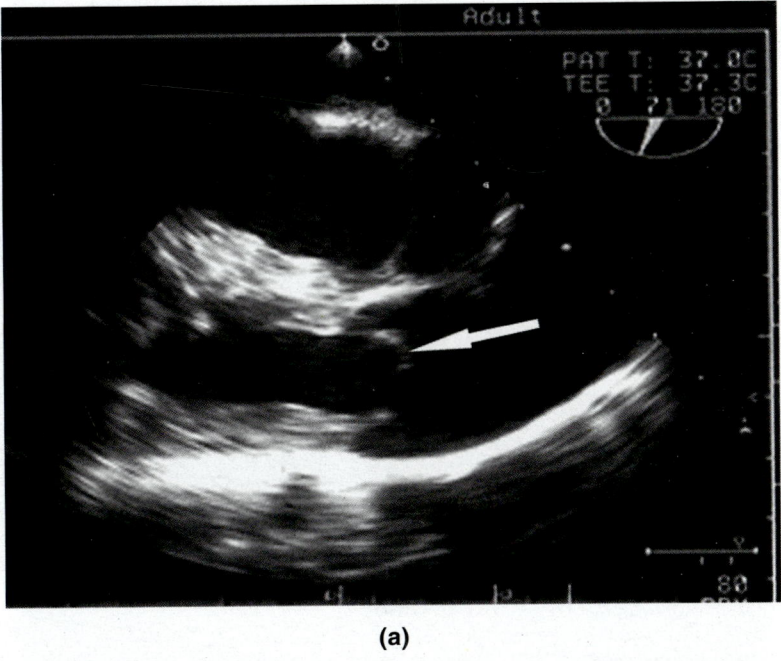

(a)

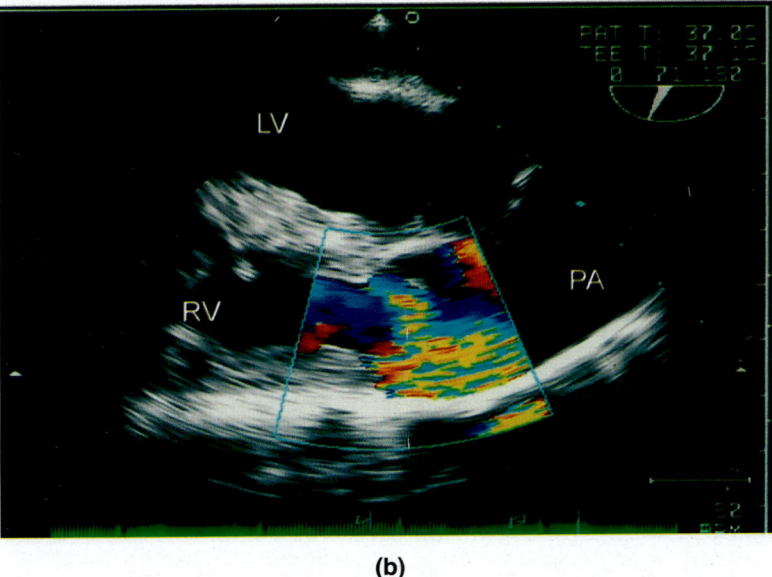

(b)

Figure 9.17. A patient with pulmonary valvular stenosis. Note the doming pulmonary valve (arrow, **a**) with turbulent flow across the valve on colour flow **(b)**. (LV : left ventricle, RV : right ventricle, PA : pulmonary artery)

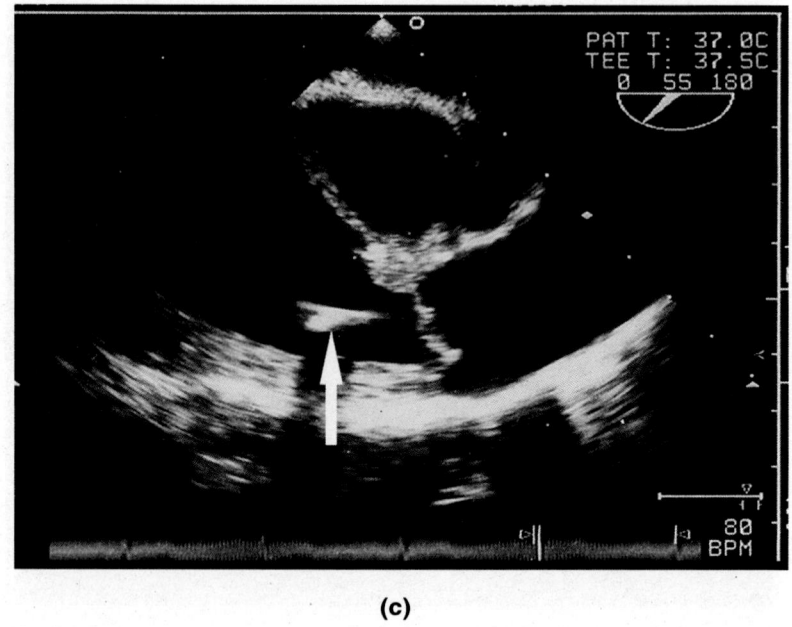

(c)

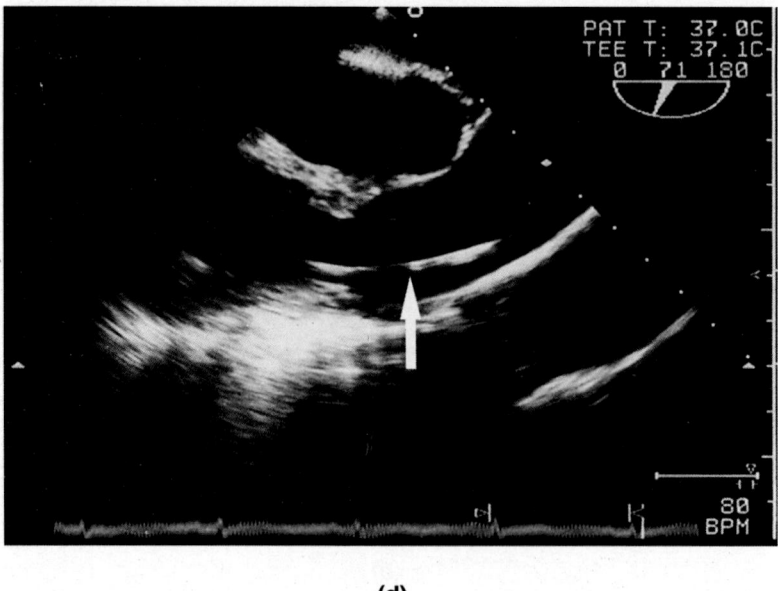

(d)

Figure 9.17 (c & d) Show a Swan-Ganz catheter (arrow, **c**) being passed across the stenosed pulmonary valve **(d)**.

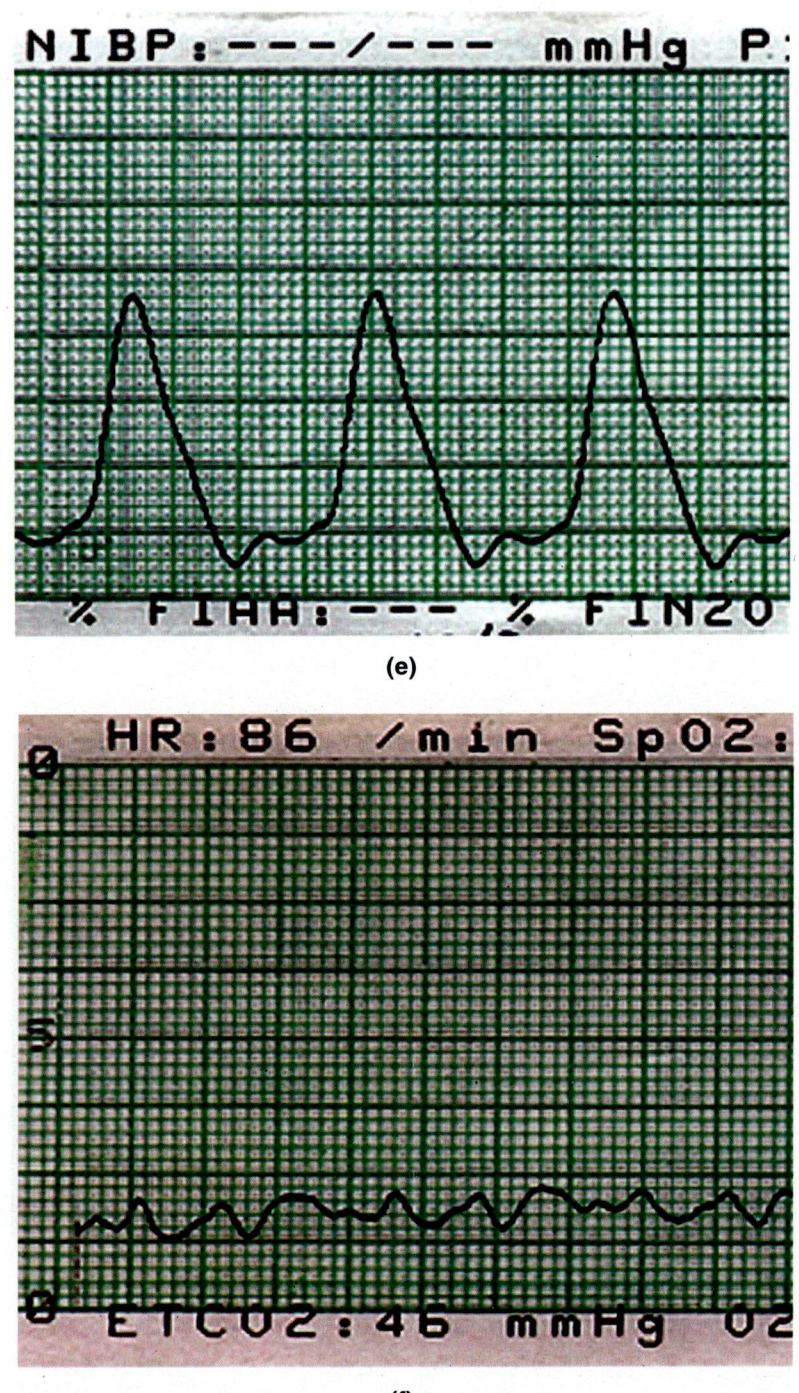

(e)

(f)

Figure 9.17 (e & f) Show pressure tracings from the same patient at right ventricular outflow **(e)** and pulmonary artery **(f)** showing a transvalvular gradient.

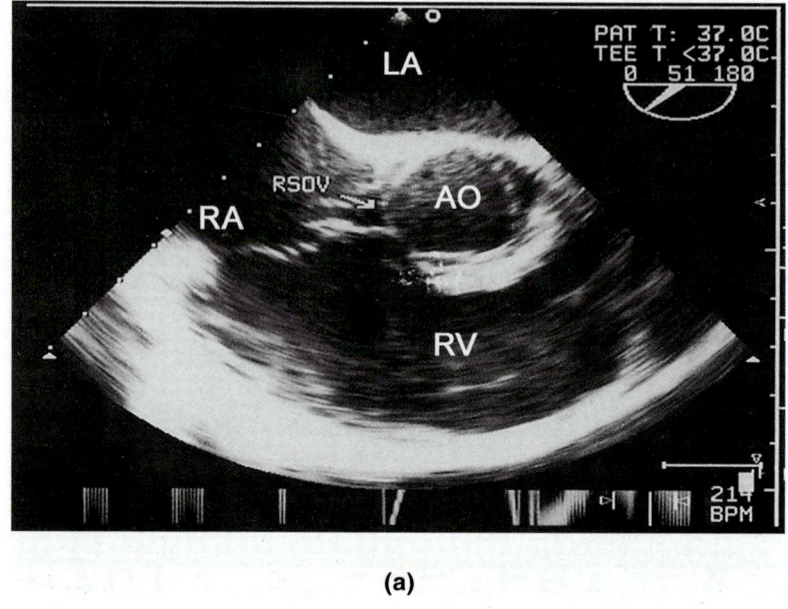

(a)

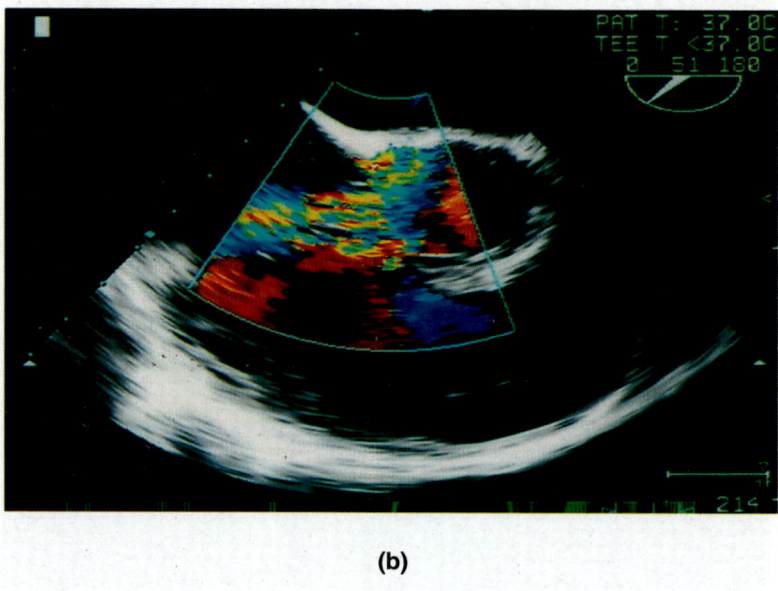

(b)

Figure 9.18 (a) Appearance of the ruptured sinus of valsalva. Note the tract arising from the aortic sinus and opening into the right atrium. **(b)** Colour flow across the fistulous tract showing a continuous shunt from the aorta to the right atrium. (LA: left atrium, RA: right atrium, RV: right ventricle, AO: aorta, RSOV: ruptured sinus of valsalva).

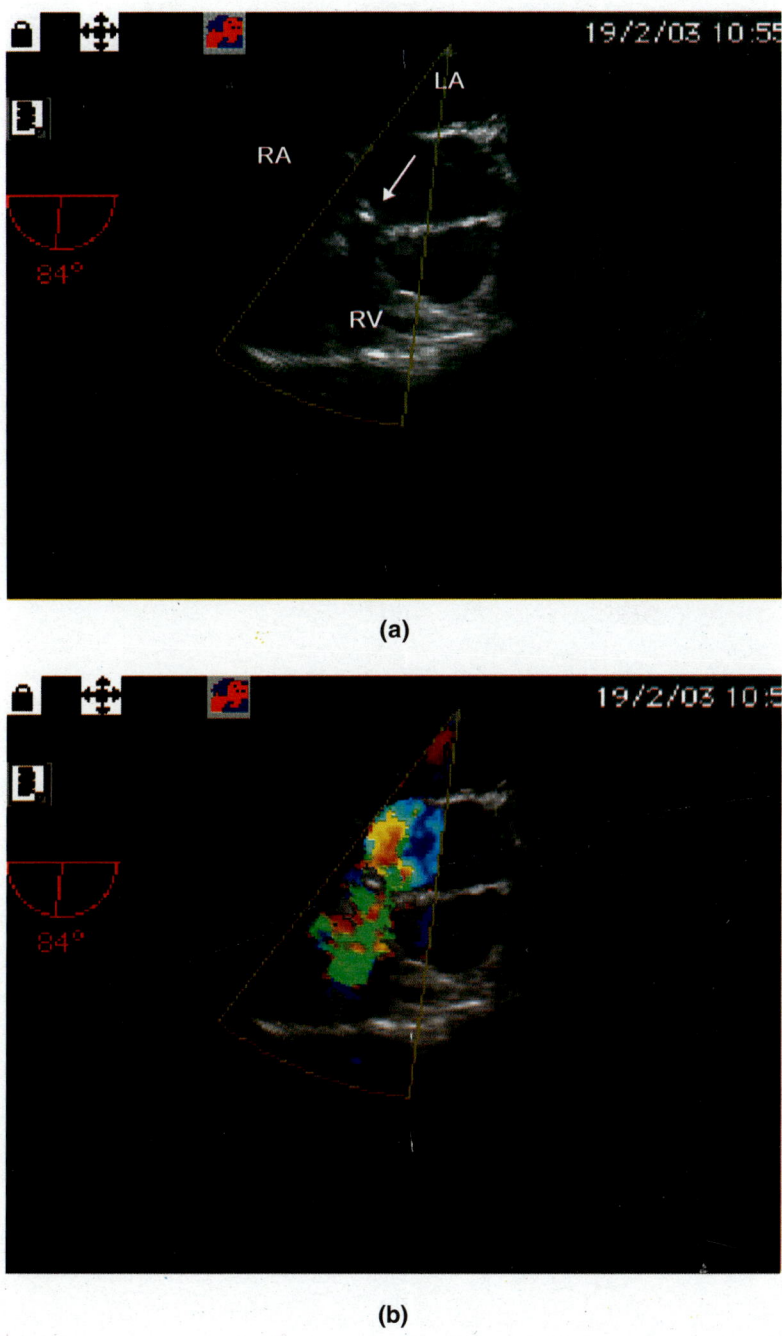

Figure 9.19 (a) Appearance of the ruptured sinus of valsalva opening into the right ventricle. Note the fistulous tract (arrow) and the dilated aortic annulus **(b)** Colour flow across the fistulous tract showing a continuous shunt from the aorta to the right ventricle. (LA: left atrium, RA: right atrium, RV: right ventricle)

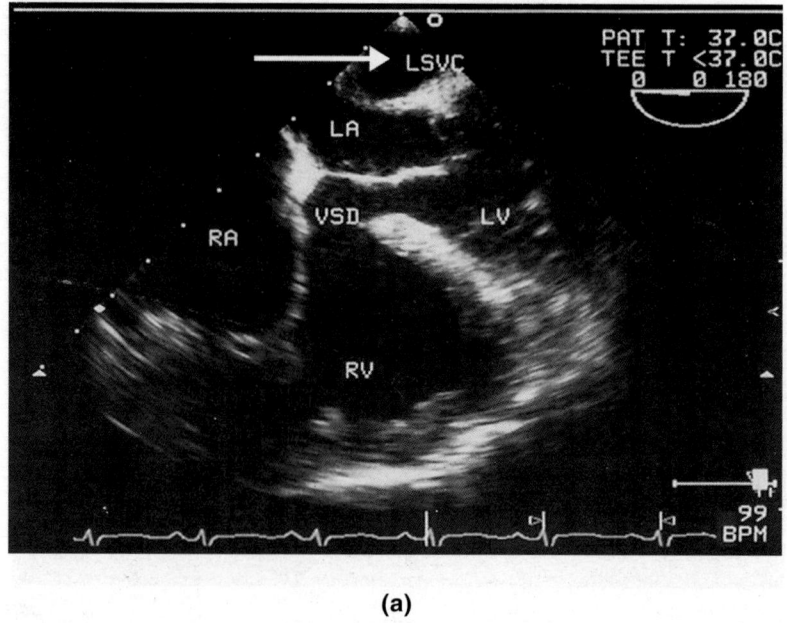

(a)

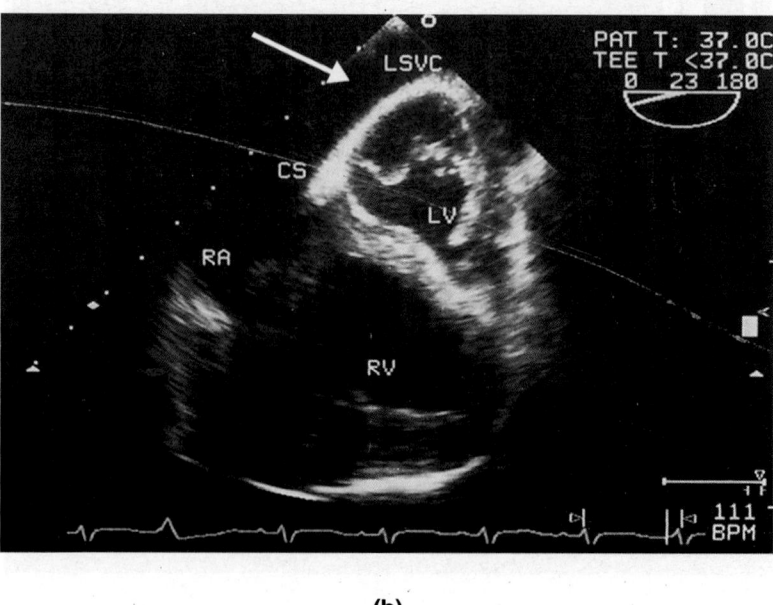

(b)

Figure 9.20 (a & b) Left superior vena cava (arrow), opening into the coronary sinus in a patient with a ventricular septal defect. (LSVC: left superior vena cava, LA: left atrium, RA: right atrium, LV: left ventricle, RV: right ventricle, VSD: ventricular septal defect, CS: coronary sinus)

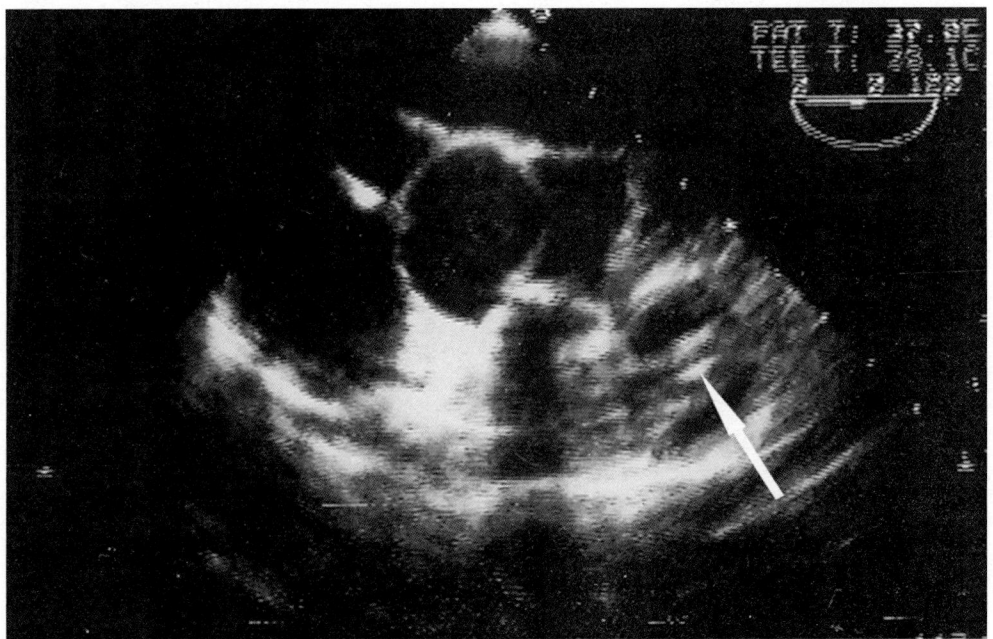

Figure 9.21. Congenital bicuspid pulmonary valve (arrow) in a patient with bicuspid aortic valve.

Chapter 10

EVALUATION OF INTRACARDIAC MASSES AND PROSTHETIC MATERIALS

The important intracardiac masses that can be visualised with trans-oesophageal echocardiography (TOE) include thrombus and tumours. Both are moderately echogenic and can be easily identified on TOE. Thrombus and tumours have different appearances with a common clinical problem of potential embolism. Those present in the venous system can cause pulmonary embolism, while those in the left heart can lead to systemic embolism. Occasionally a right sided thrombus / tumour can embolise into the systemic circulation via intracardiac defects such as atrial or ventricular septal defects.

Thrombus formation is related to stagnant blood flow, which depicts a spontaneous echo contrast. Left atrial thrombus is predominantly found in patients with mitral stenosis and /or atrial fibrillation due to stagnation of blood in the left atrium. The spontaneous echo contrast is seen in a dilated left atrium showing slow whirling movement. Left atrial appendage is the most common site of thrombus formation, but can also be found in the body or the posterior wall of the left atrium. Left ventricular thrombus is often associated with myocardial infarction or left ventricular aneurysm. Pulmonary thrombus is generally the result of embolism from the veins of the pelvis and lower extremities.

The most common primary tumour of the heart is myxoma. It is pathologically benign, but is fragile and can cause systemic embolism. It appears as a soft and mobile mass on TOE. The left atrial myxoma is more common than the right atrial myxoma with an attachment to the interatrial septum. The mobile tumour in the left atrium can occlude the mitral valve opening during diastole leading to symptoms of mitral stenosis.

In this chapter, atrial myxomas of various shapes and sizes visualised in different views have been shown. Likewise, the appearance of atrial and venticular thrombi in different views have been illustrated. TOE can also be utilised to visualise the correct placement of the pulmonary artery catheter and intracardiac cannulae by the surgeon. Images illustrating their appearance have also been included.

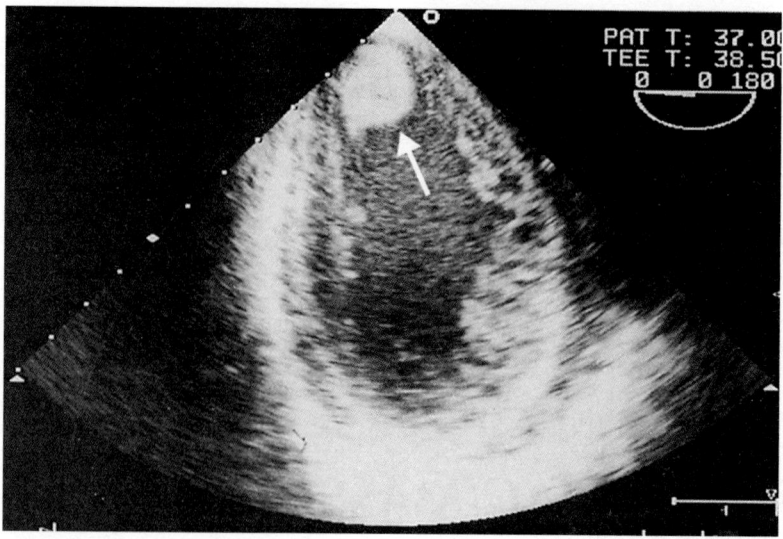

Figure 10.1. Transgastric short axis view of the left ventricle in a patient with inferior wall myocardial infarction. Note the aneurysm in the inferior wall with a clot (arrow).

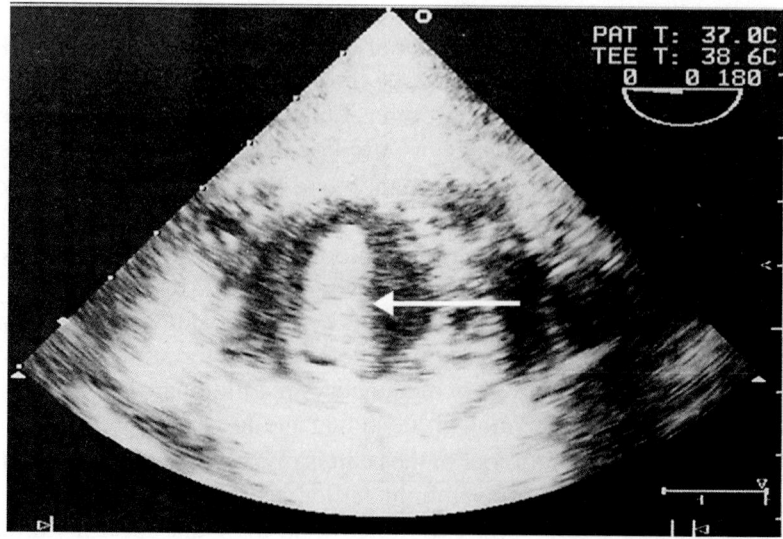

Figure 10.2. A patient with anterior wall myocardial infarction and an apical aneurysm. Trans-gastric short axis view of the left ventricle showing a clot near the apex (arrow).

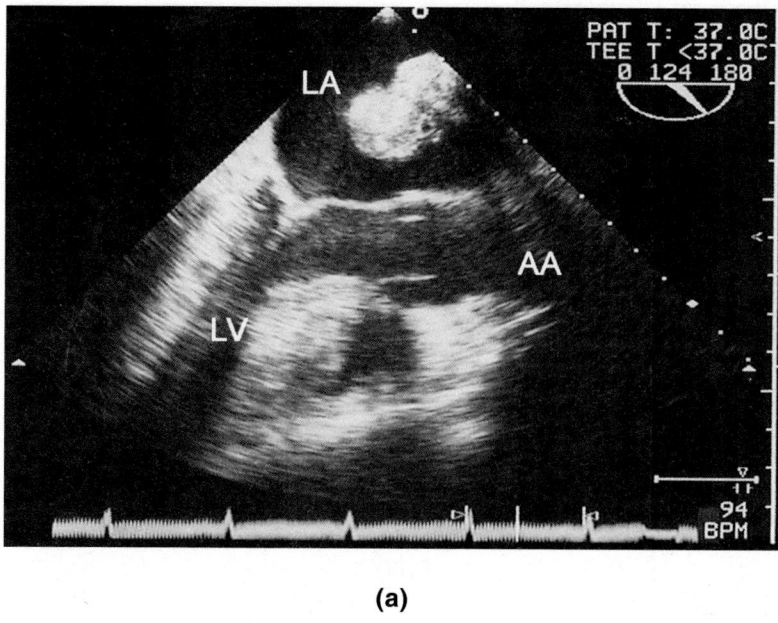

(a)

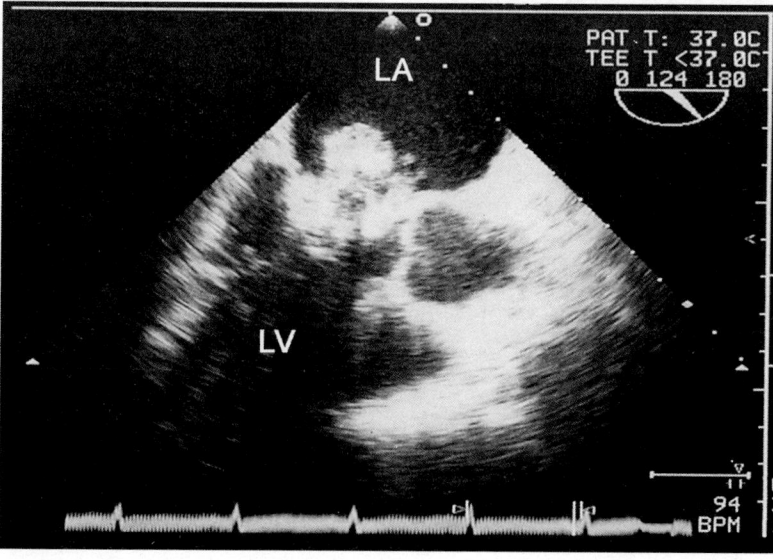

(b)

Figure 10.3. A mobile left atrial myxoma. Note the to and fro movement of the myxoma in the left atrium in systole **(a)** and diastole **(b)** causing mitral valve obstruction. (LA: left atrium, LV: left ventricle, AA: ascending aorta)

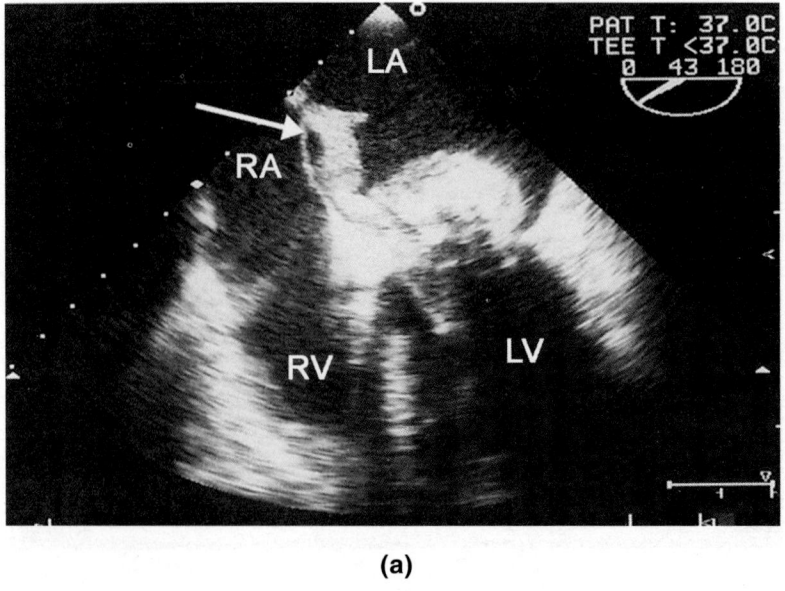

(a)

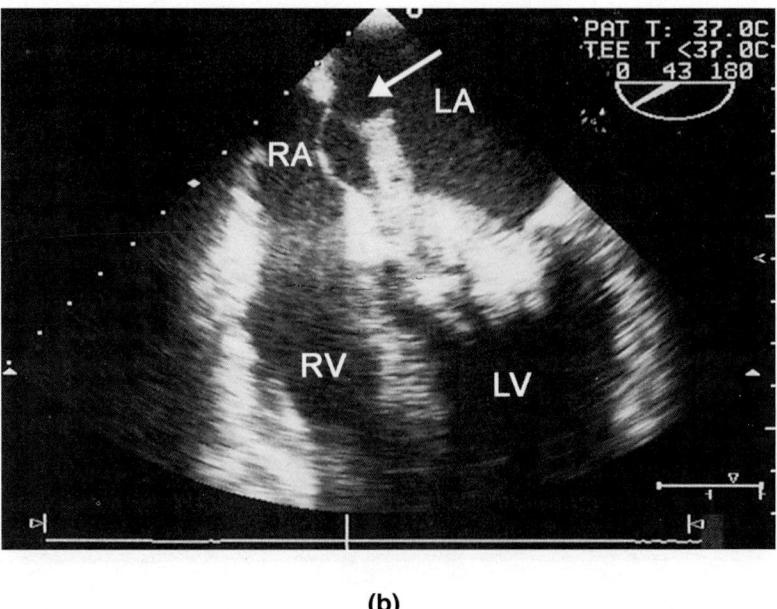

(b)

Figure 10.4 (a & b) A large left atrial myxoma obstructing the mitral valve. Note the peduncle (arrow) of the myxoma arising from the inter-atrial septum. (LA: Left atrium, LV: left ventricle, RA: right atrium, RV: right ventricle)

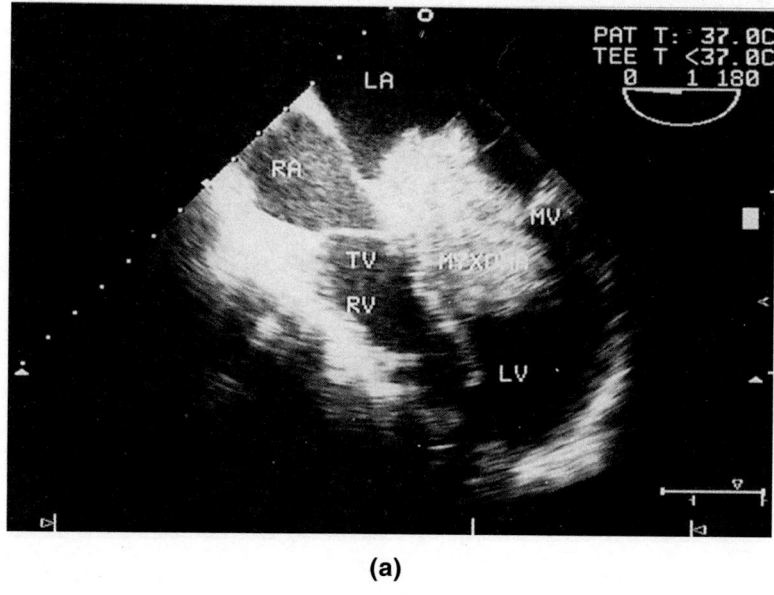

(a)

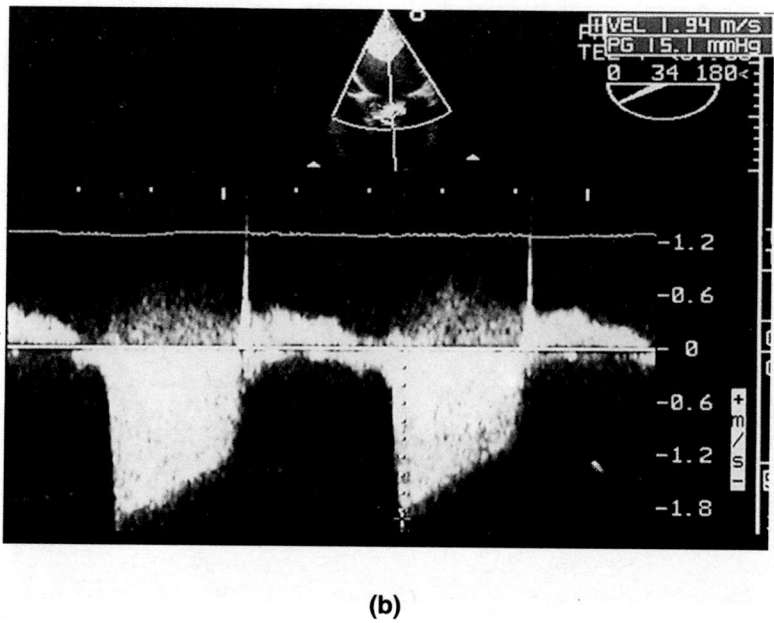

(b)

Figure 10.5 (a) A large left atrial myxoma prolapsing across the mitral valve. **(b)** Note the continuous wave Doppler across the mitral valve showing a large transmitral gradient. (LA: left atrium, RA: right atrium, RV: right ventricle, LV: left ventricle, TV: tricuspid valve, MV: mitral valve)

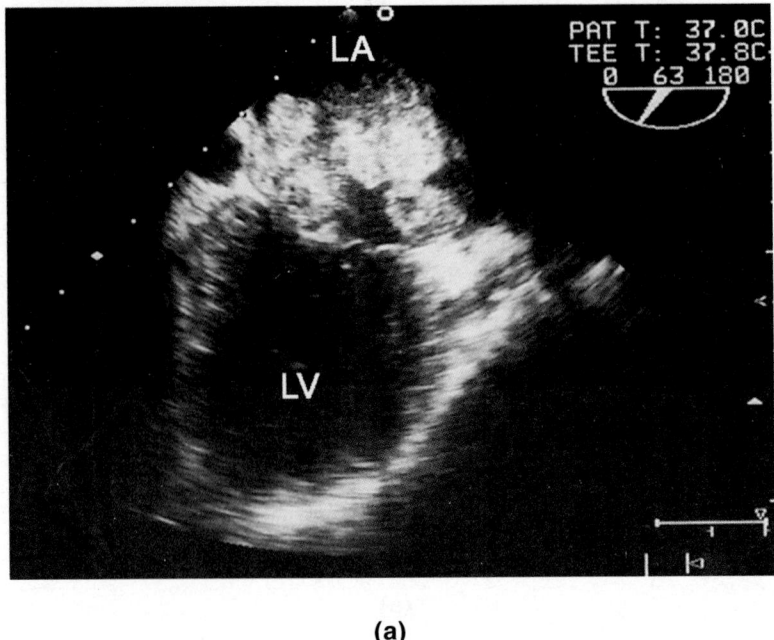

(a)

(b)

Figure 10.6 (a) Two chamber view showing a fragile left atrial myxoma with a variegated appearance. **(b)** Short axis transgastric view in the same patient showing a portion of the myxoma prolapsing into the left ventricle. (LA: left atrium, LV: left ventricle)

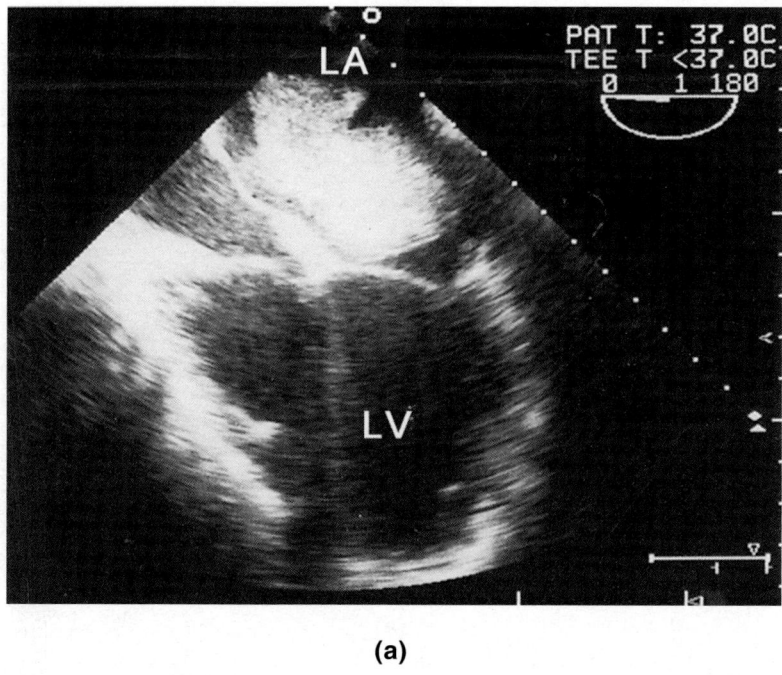

(a)

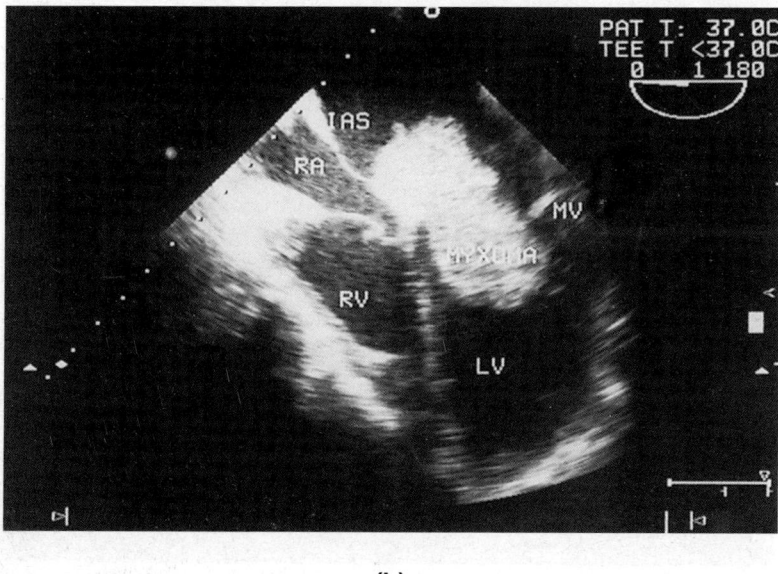

(b)

Figure 10.7. Mobile large left atrial myxoma. Note the two and fro motion across the mitral valve in systole **(a)** and diastole **(b)** (RA: right atrium, RV: right ventricle, LV: left ventricle, IAS: inter-atrial septum, MV: mitral valve)

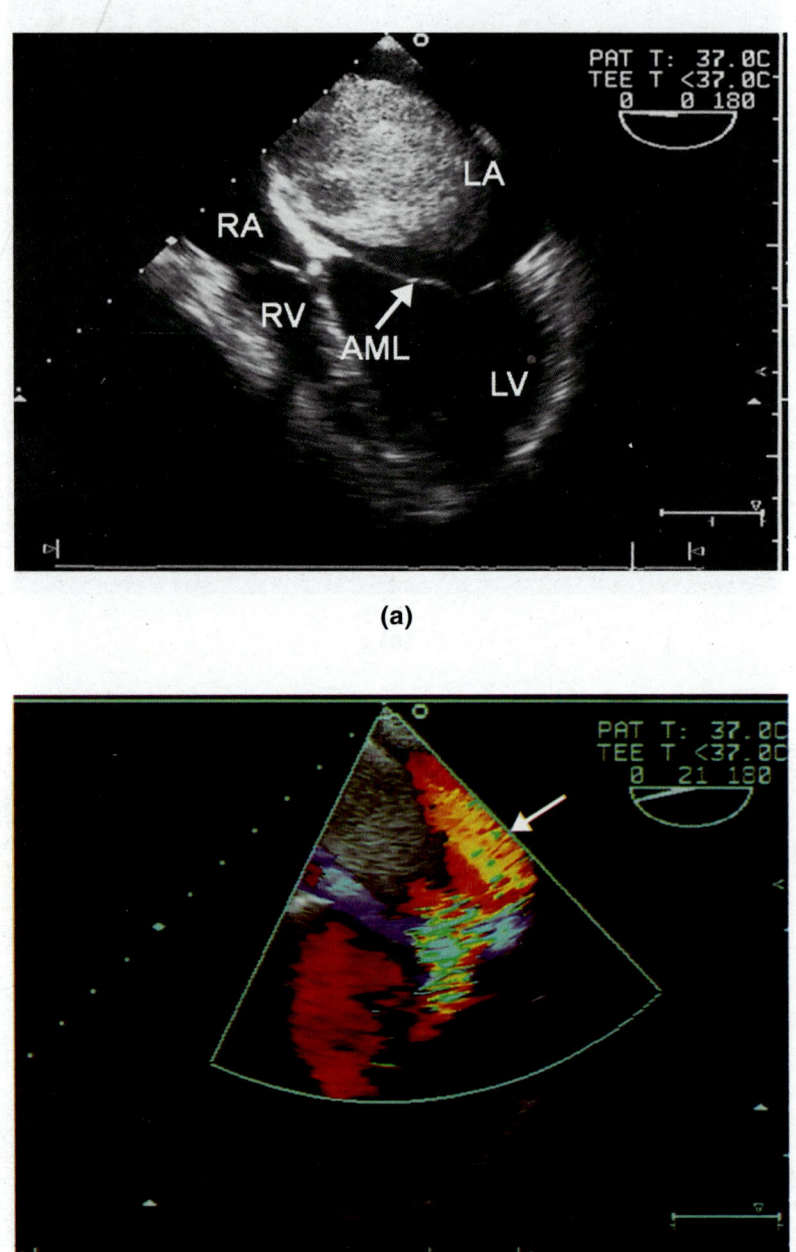

(a)

(b)

Figure 10.8 (a) A large left atrial myxoma arising from the inter-atrial septum and projecting over the anterior mitral leaflet (AML). **(b)** Note the mitral regurgitant jet (arrow) resulting from improper coaptation of the mitral leaflets. (LA: left atrium, RA: right atrium, RV: right ventricle, LV: left ventricle)

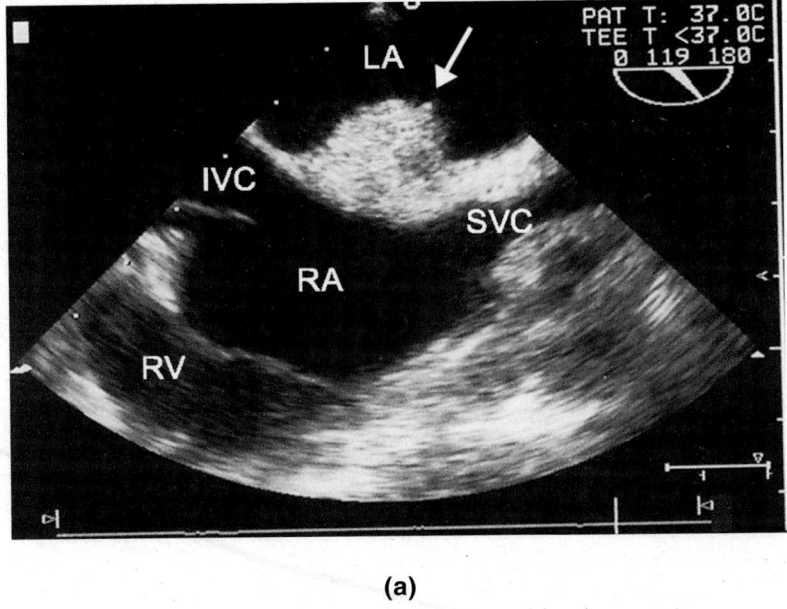

(a)

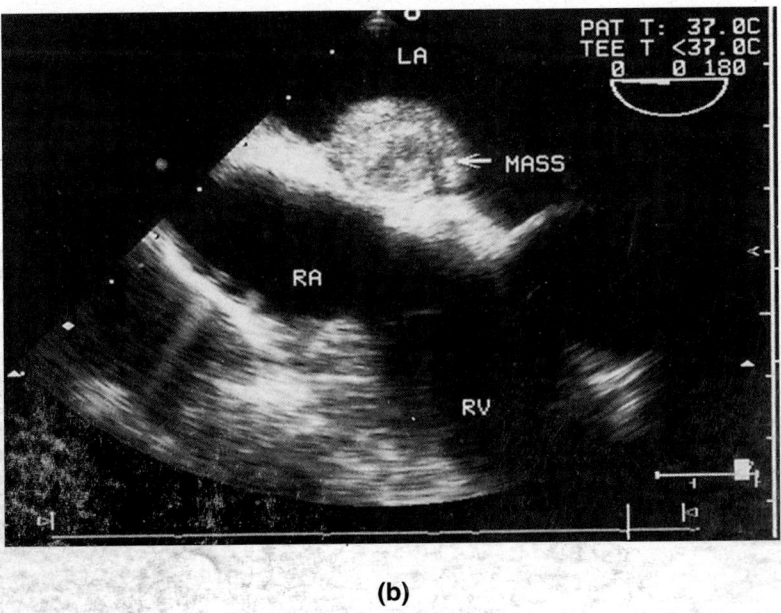

(b)

Figure 10.9. Small left atrial myxoma (arrow) arising from the inter-atrial septum.
(a) bicaval view, **(b)** four chamber view. (LA: left atrium, RA: right atrium, RV: right ventricle, SVC: superior vena cava, IVC: inferior vena cava)

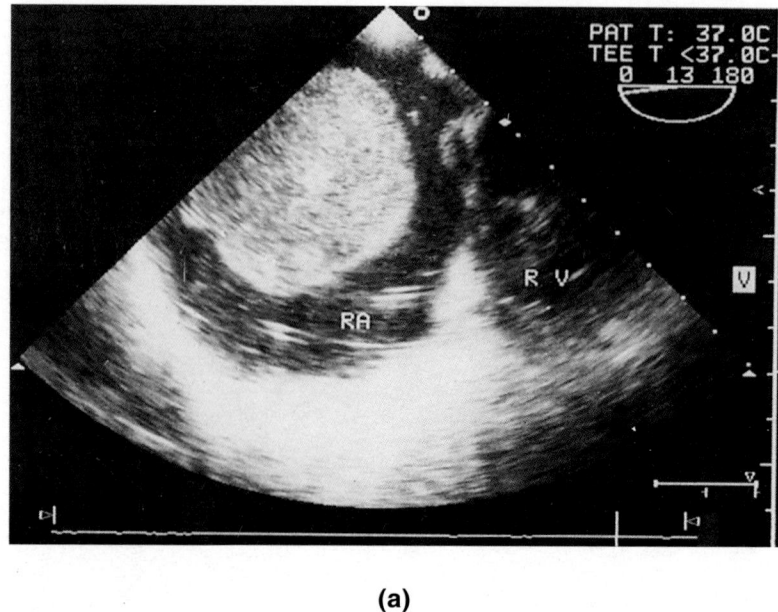

(a)

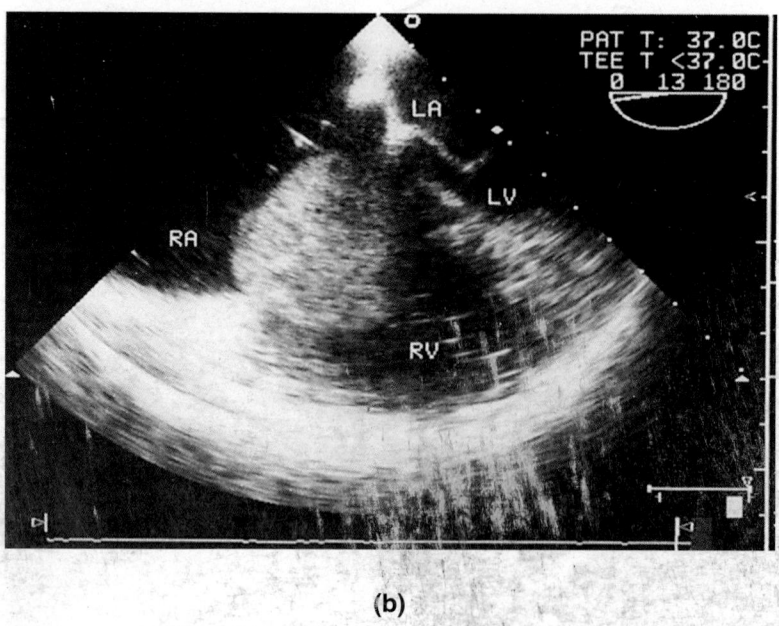

(b)

Figure 10.10 (a & b) A large right atrial myxoma prolapsing across the tricuspid valve. (LA: left atrium, RA: right atrium, RV: right ventricle, LV: left ventricle)

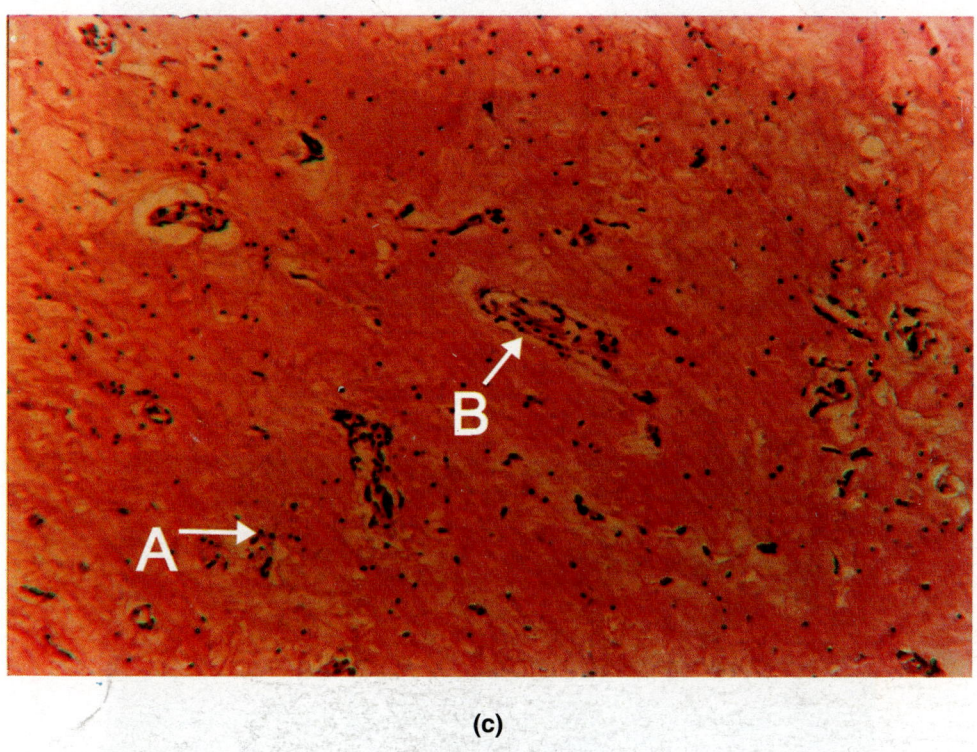

(c)

Figure 10.10 (c) Histopathologic appearance of the right atrial myxoma showing stellate to polyhedral cells seen in clusters (arrow A) or single cells in a loose myxoid stroma. These features characteristic of a myxoma are more prominent around the vascular spaces (arrow B). (H&E x 100)

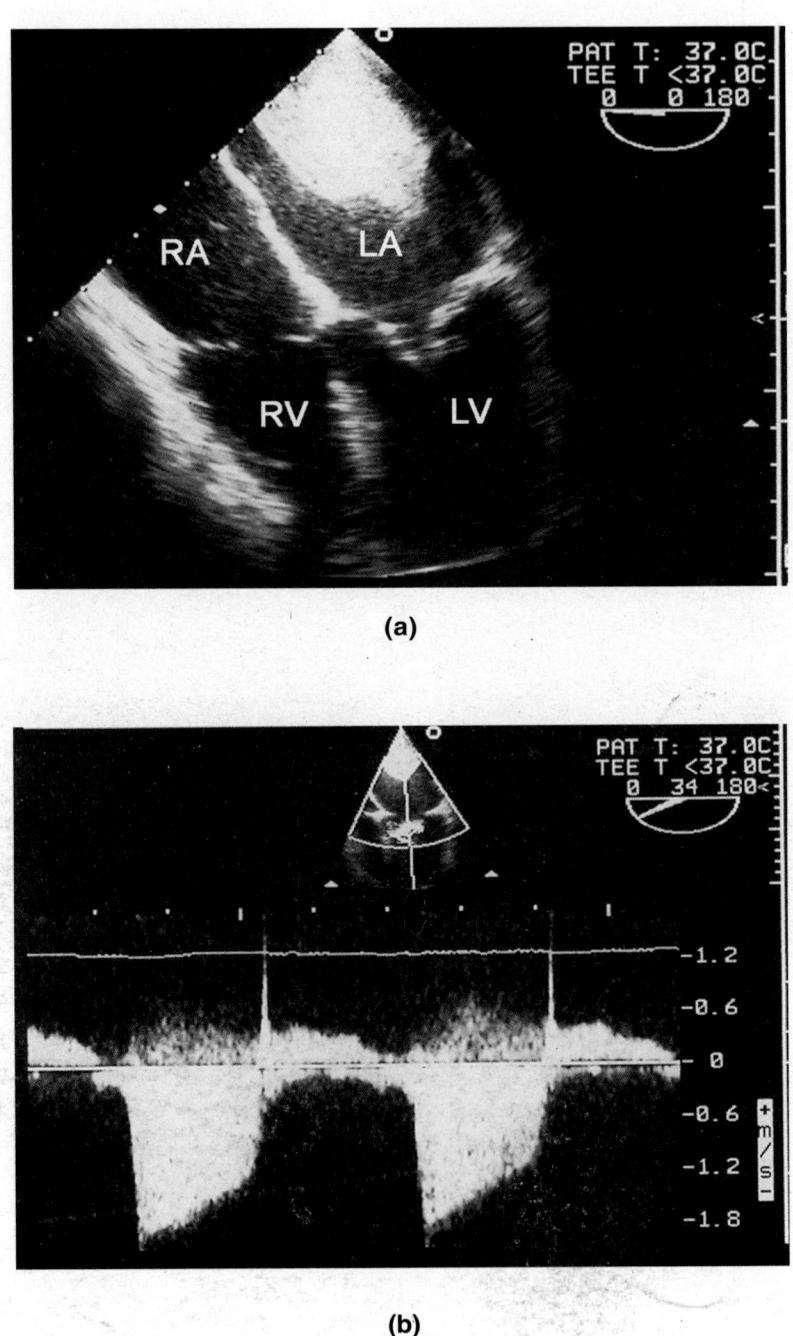

(a)

(b)

Figure 10.11 (a) Four chamber view showing a large left atrial clot in a patient with rheumatic mitral stenosis. **(b)** Trans-mitral continuous wave Doppler in the same patient showed a peak gradient of 14 mm Hg and mean gradient of 9 mm Hg. (RA: right atrium, LA: left atrium, RV: right ventricle, LV: left ventricle)

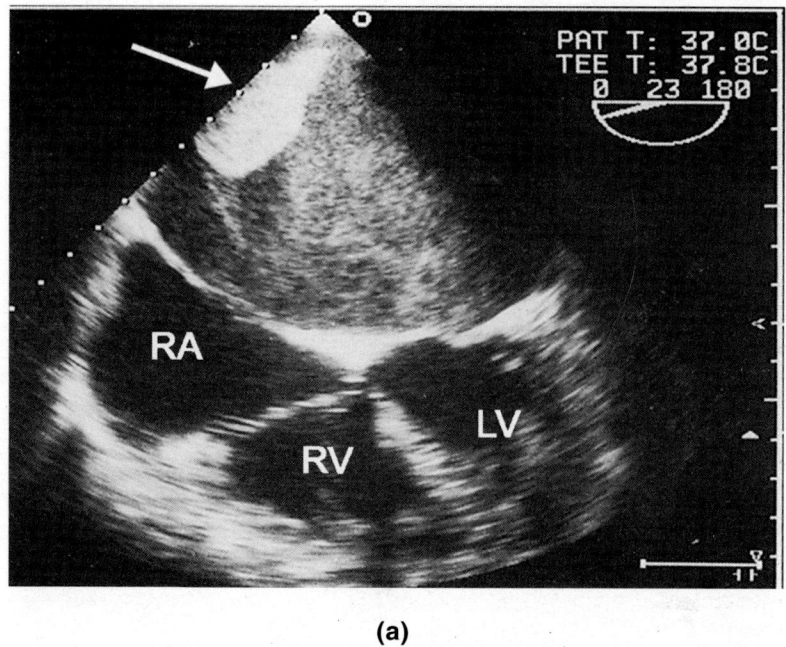

(a)

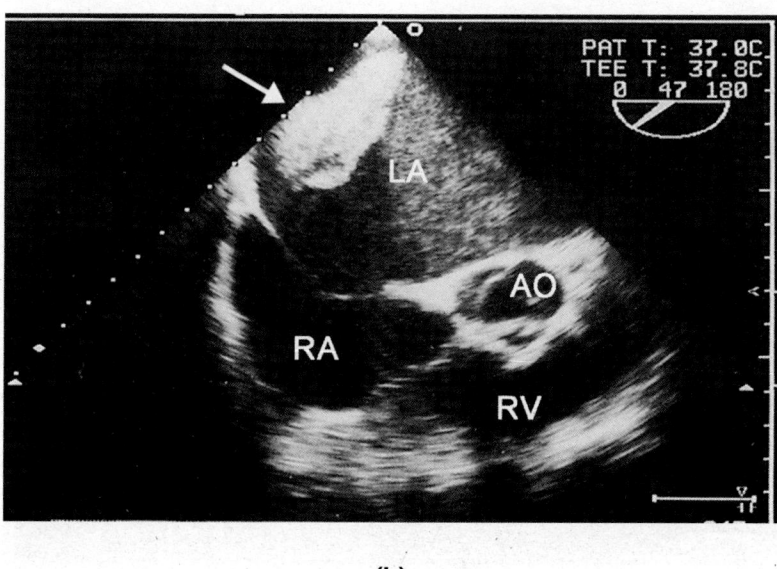

(b)

Figure 10.12 (a & b) Spontaneous echo contrast and left atrial body clot (arrow) in a patient with rheumatic mitral stenosis. (LA: left atrium, RA: right atrium, RV: right ventricle, LV: left ventricle, AO: aorta)

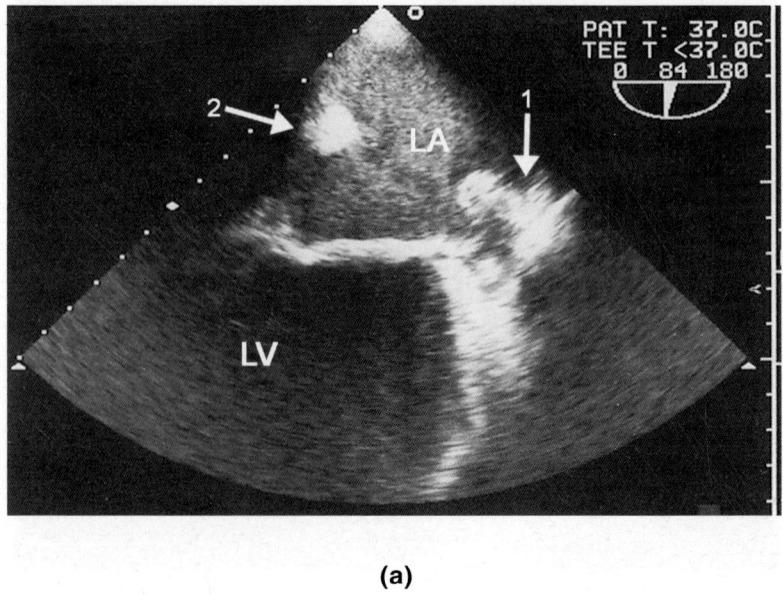

(a)

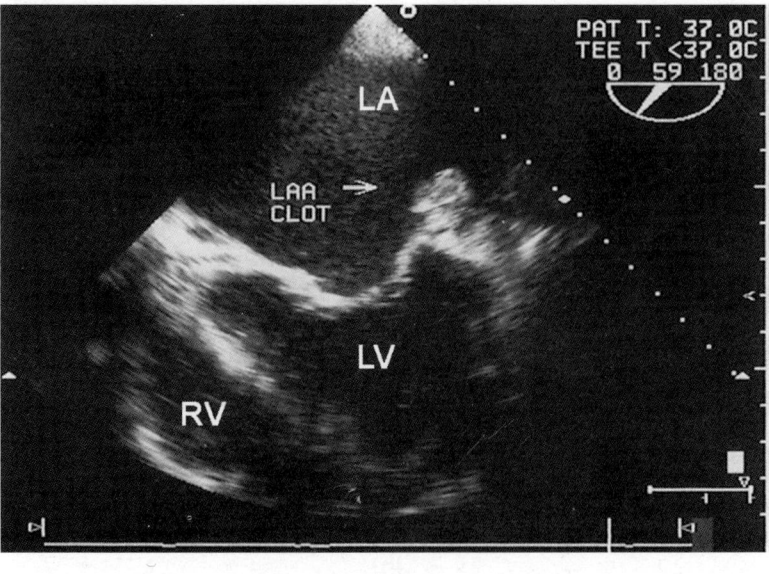

(b)

Figure 10.13 (a & b) Left atrial appendage clot (arrow 1) and left atrial body clot (arrow 2) in a patient with severe mitral stenosis. (LA: left atrium, LV: left ventricle, RV: right ventricle, LAA : left atrial appendage)

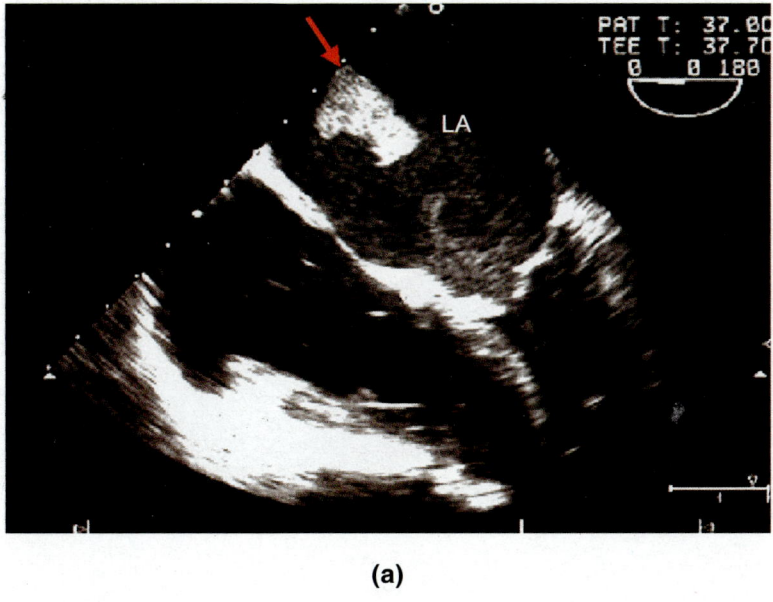

(a)

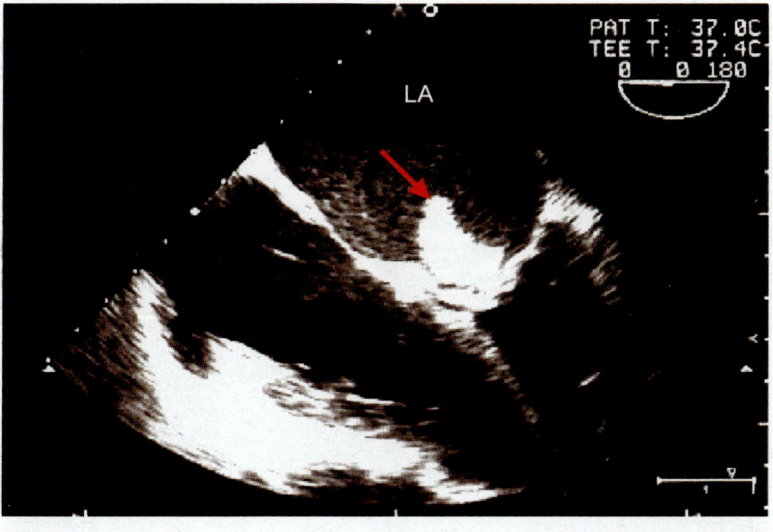

(b)

Figure 10.14. Mobile floating thrombus (ping pong motion) in a patient with severe mitral stenosis. **(a)** At the onset of diastole mass is deep in left atrial cavity, **(b)** mass moves with antegrade transmitral flow in diastole but cannot cross mitral valve due to severe stenosis. (LA: Left atrium)

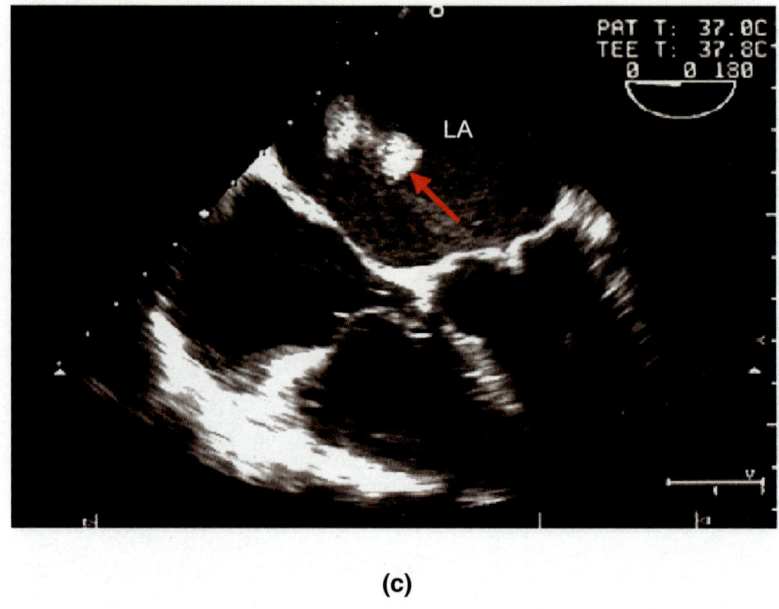

(c)

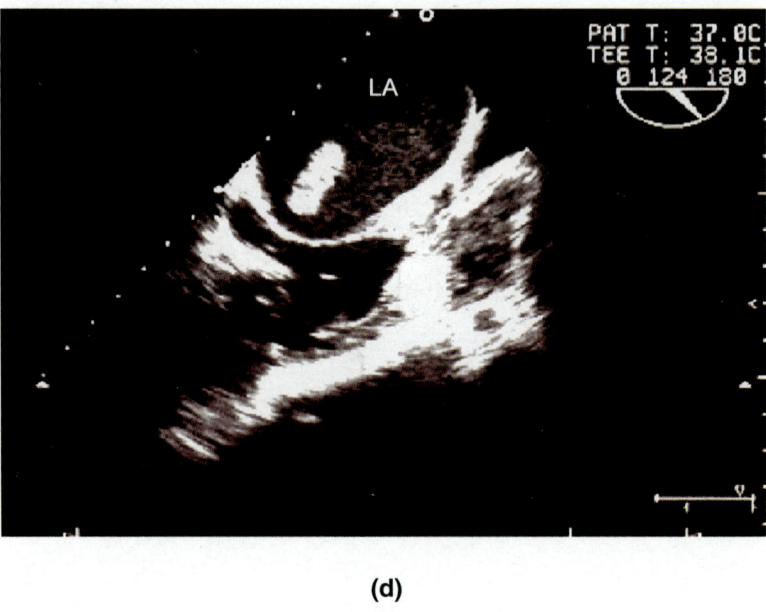

(d)

Figure 10.14 (c) In systole the mitral valve closes and hits the mass causing it to move back again deep in left atrial cavity, **(d)** upper oesophageal view (124º) in the same patient. (LA: Left atrium)

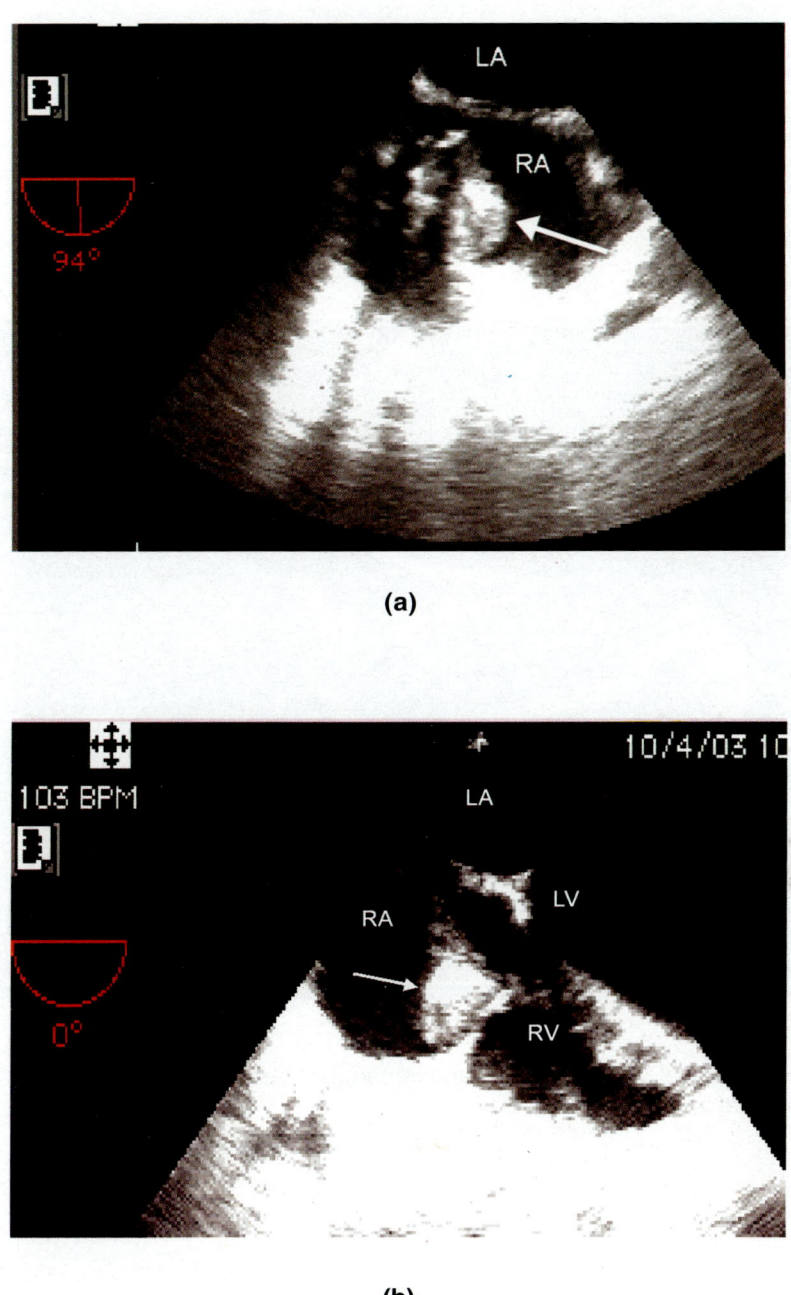

Figure 10.15. Right atrial mass (arrow) in bicaval view **(a)** and 4 chamber view **(b)**. Echocardiographic appearance of such a mass may not always be diagnostic for differentiating myxoma from a thrombus. Histopathology in this case revealed the mass to be a thrombus. (LA: left atrium, RA: right atrium, LV: left ventricle, RV: right ventricle)

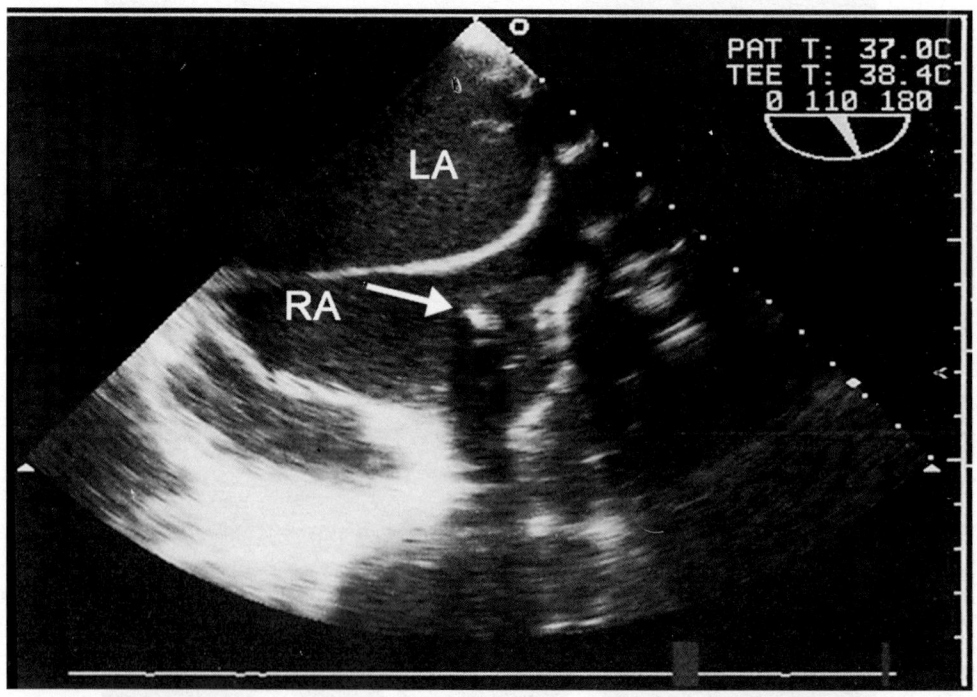

Figure 10.16. Bicaval view showing venous cannula (arrow) in the right atrium. (LA: left atrium, RA: right atrium)

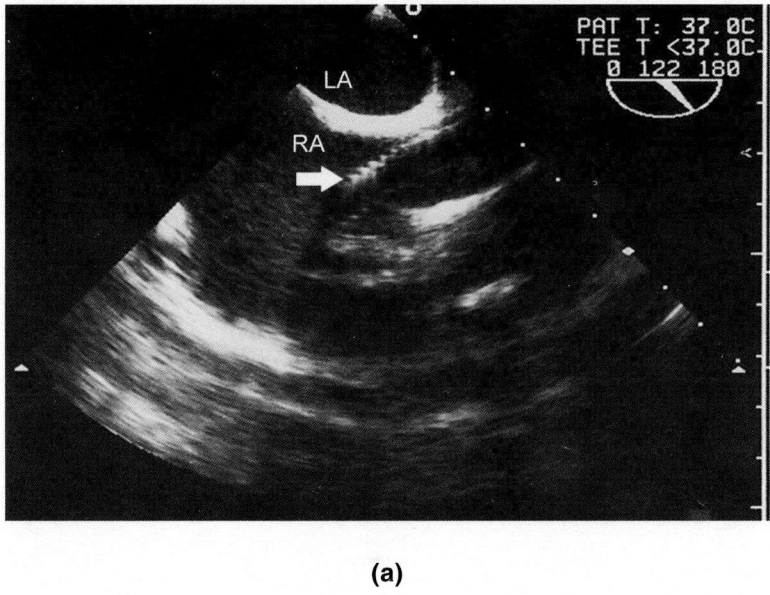

(a)

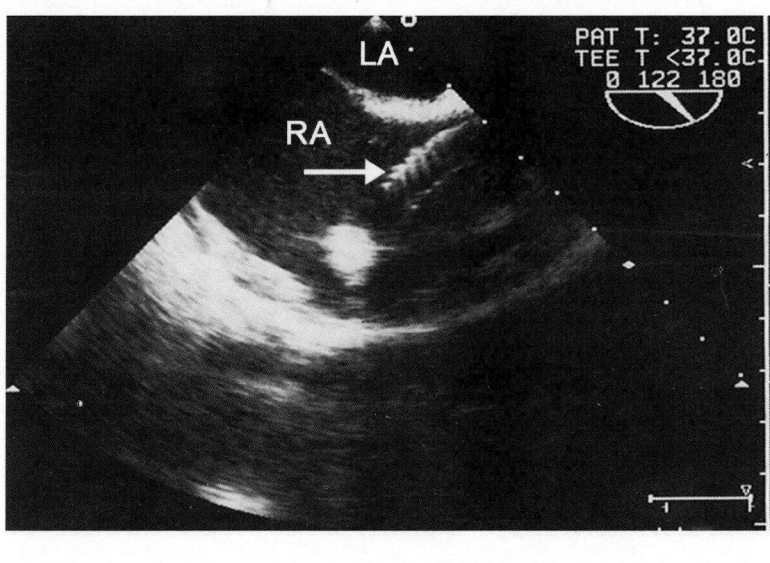

(b)

Figure 10.17 (a and b) Bicaval view showing venous cannula (arrow) directed in the superior vena cava. (LA: left atrium, RA: right atrium)

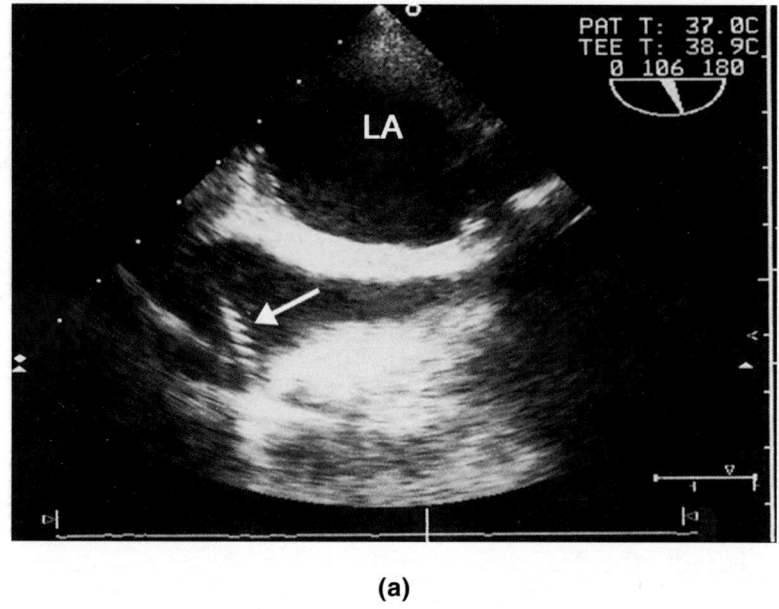

(a)

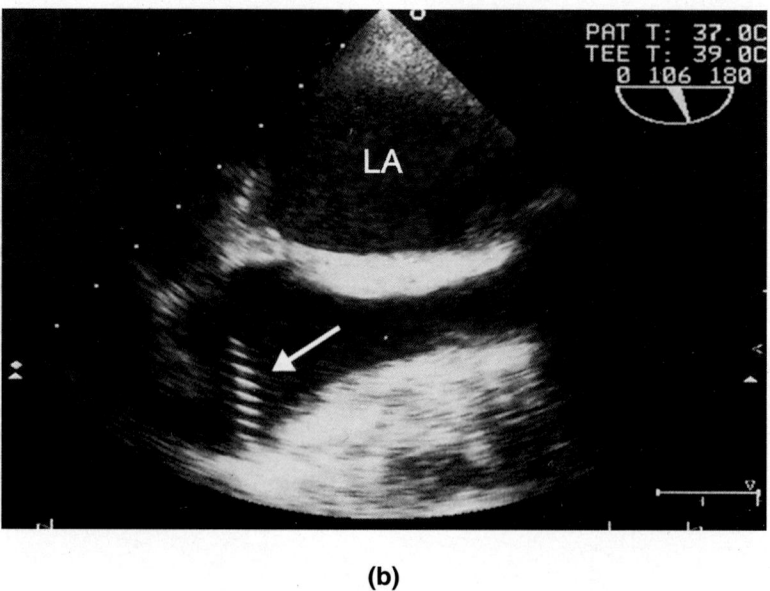

(b)

Figure 10.18 (a and b) Bicaval view showing venous cannula (arrow) directed in the inferior vena cava. (LA: left atrium)

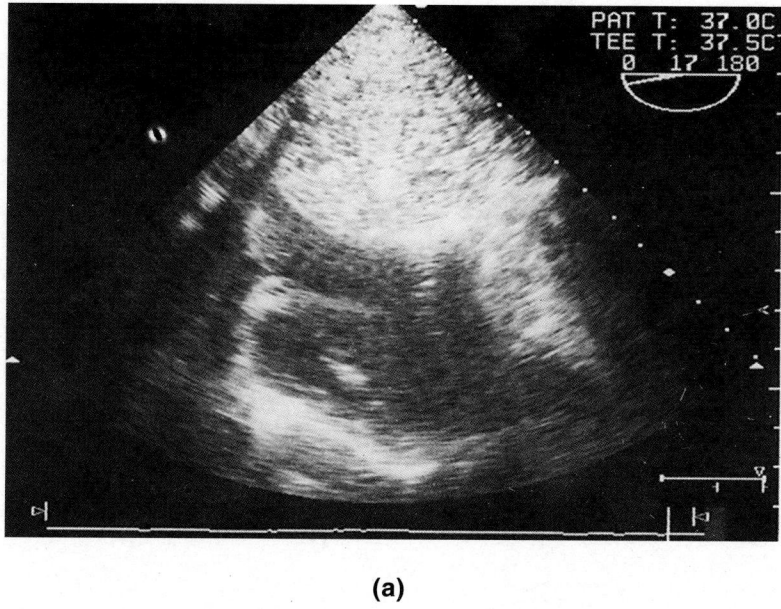

(a)

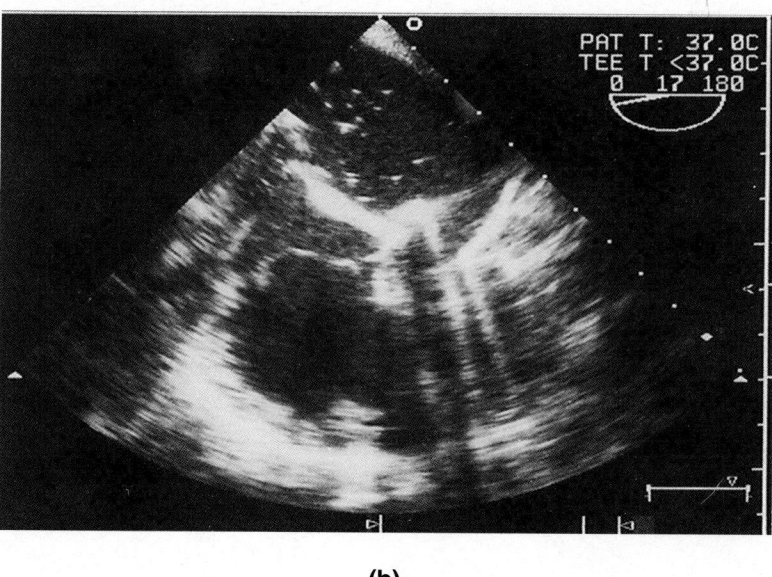

(b)

Figure 10.19. Use of trans-oesophageal echo for confirming adequate de-airing before release of aortic clamp for preventing systemic air embolism. Note large quantity of air in the left atrium in a patient who underwent mitral valve replacement **(a)**. Adequate de-airing was subsequently confirmed before releasing the aortic cross clamp **(b)**.

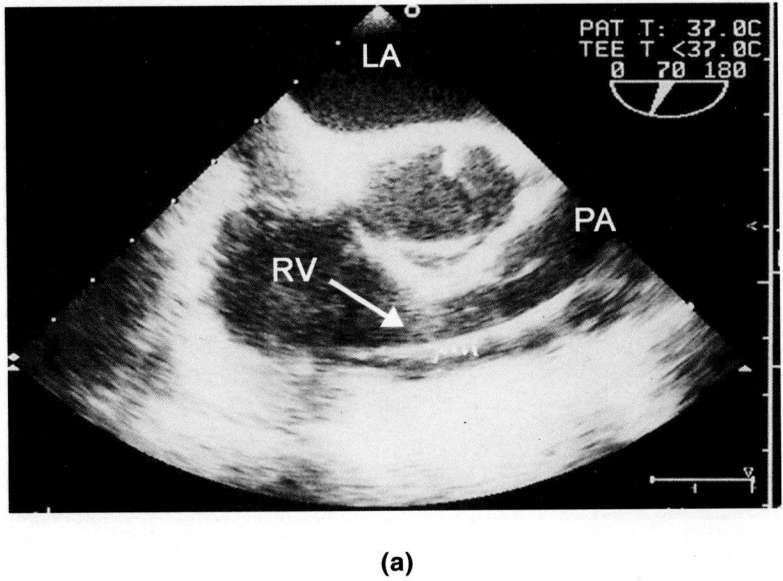

(a)

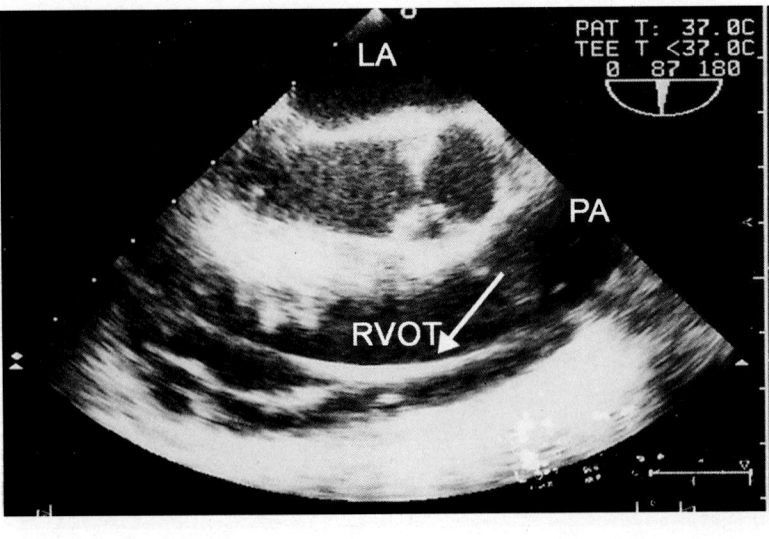

(b)

Figure 10.20 (a & b) Appearance of catheter (arrow) placed peroperatively for recording pulmonary artery pressures. (LA: left atrium, RV: right ventricle, PA: pulmonary artery, RVOT: right ventricular outflow tract)

Chapter 11

EVALUATION OF THE AORTA

Examination of the thoracic aorta with trans-oesophageal echocardiography (TOE) is an important aspect during the operative period. The examination of the ascending aorta especially with the view to detect the atheromas is important in patients undergoing coronary artery bypass grafting. The detection of atheromas can help to alter the surgical techniques so that the manipulation of the aorta is avoided. Thereby, the risk of systemic embolisation (in particular cerebral) can be prevented. TOE is also an important tool for the diagnosis of the dissection of the ascending aorta.

This chapter depicts the appearance of the normal aorta in different views. It also shows the appearance of the atheromas and dissection of the aorta.

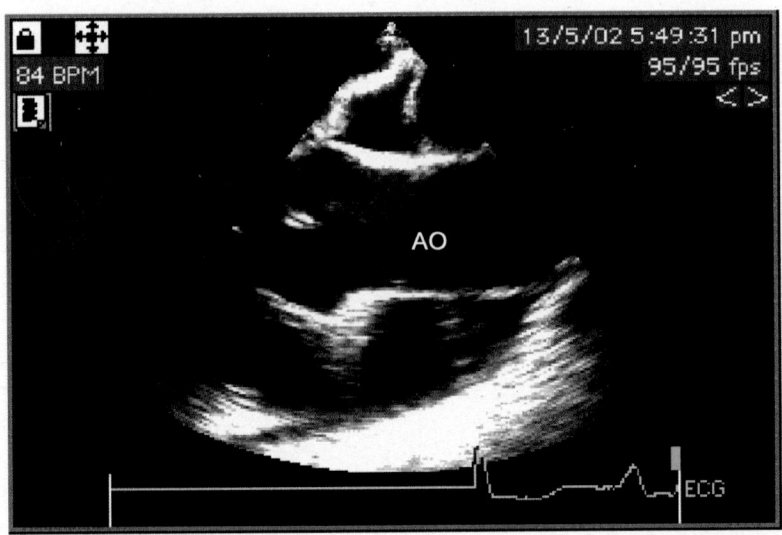

Figure 11.1. Use of upper oesophageal view for examining ascending thoracic aorta (AO).

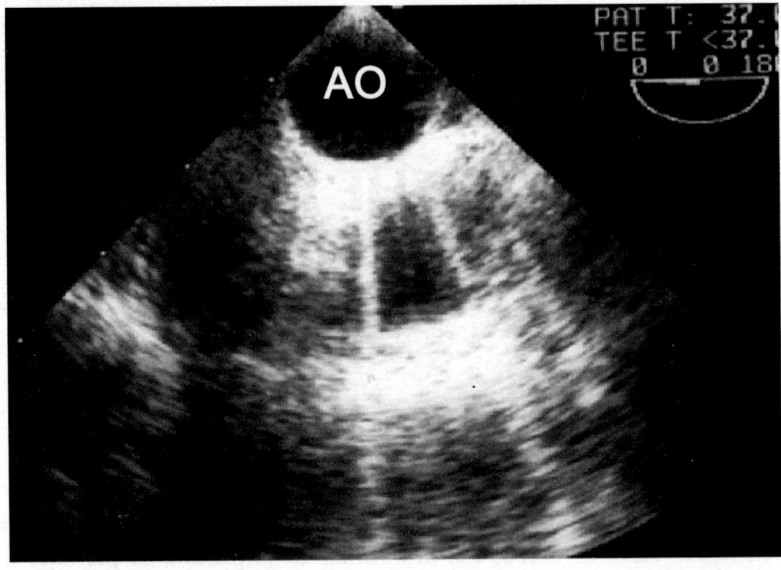

Figure 11.2. Mid-oesophageal short axis view for examining descending thoracic aorta (AO).

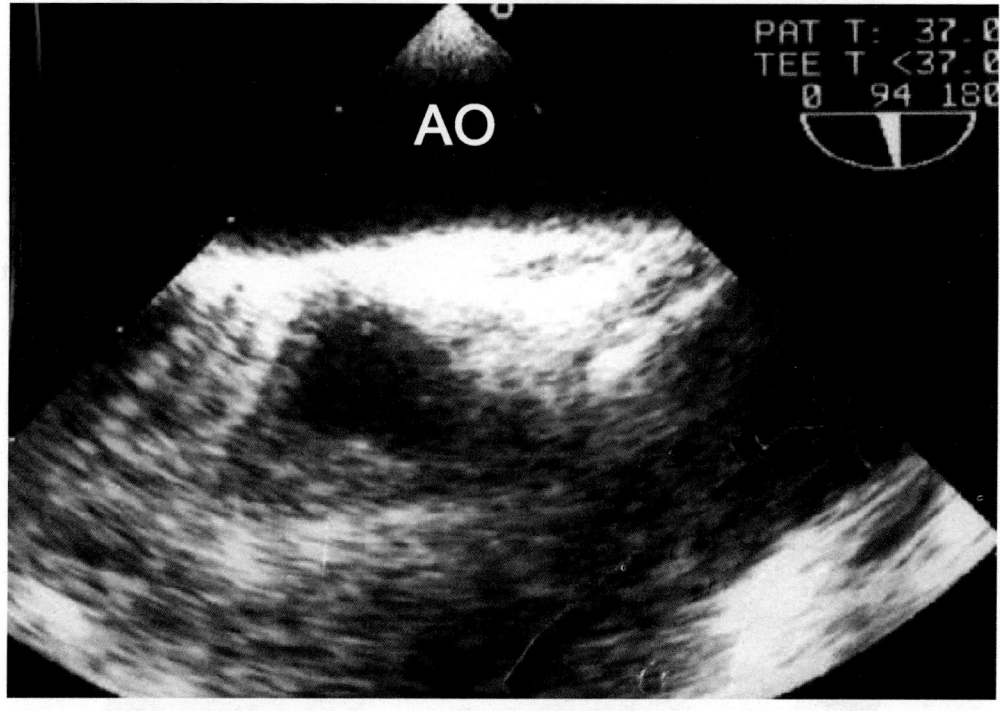

Figure 11.3. Use of mid-oesophageal view for assessing descending thoracic aorta (AO) in its long axis.

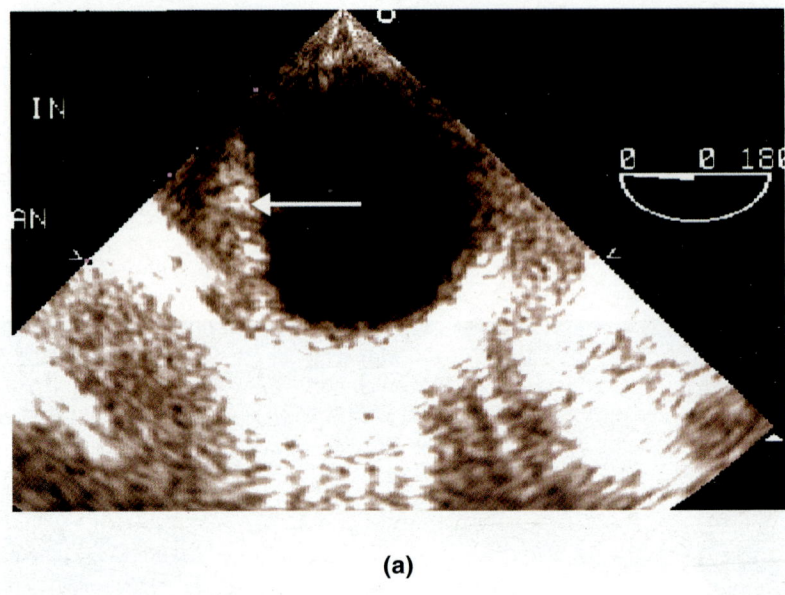

(a)

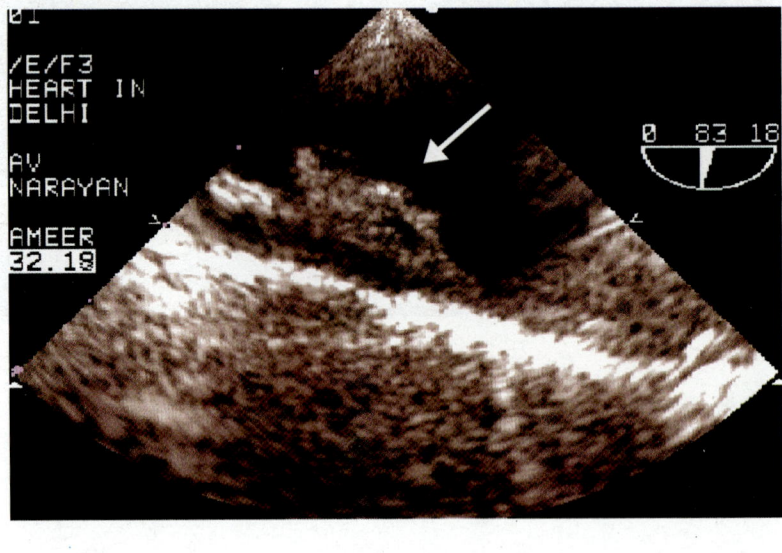

(b)

Figure 11.4. Intraoperative detection of a large aortic atheroma in descending thoracic aorta (arrow) in short axis **(a)** and long-axis **(b)**. Atherosclerotic lesions of aorta constitute a major cause of perioperative peripheral embolism and ischaemic events.

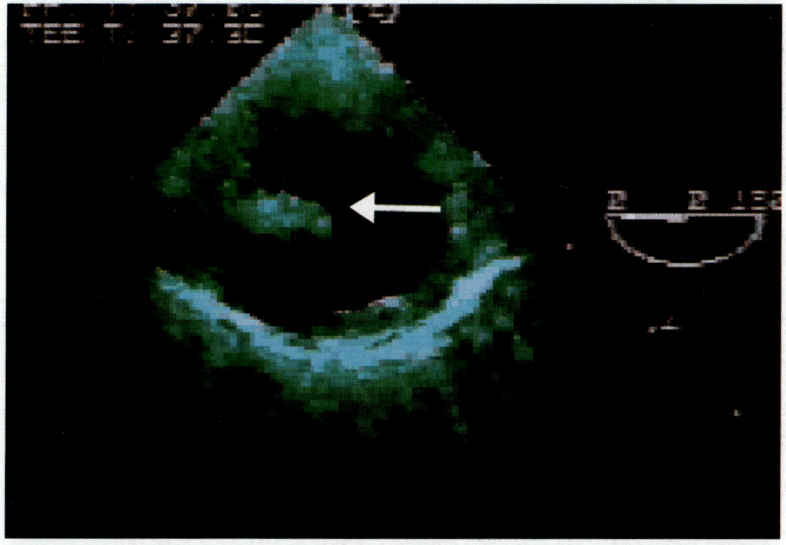

Figure 11.5. Intraoperative trans-oesophageal echocardiogram showing a large projecting aortic atheroma in the descending thoracic aorta.

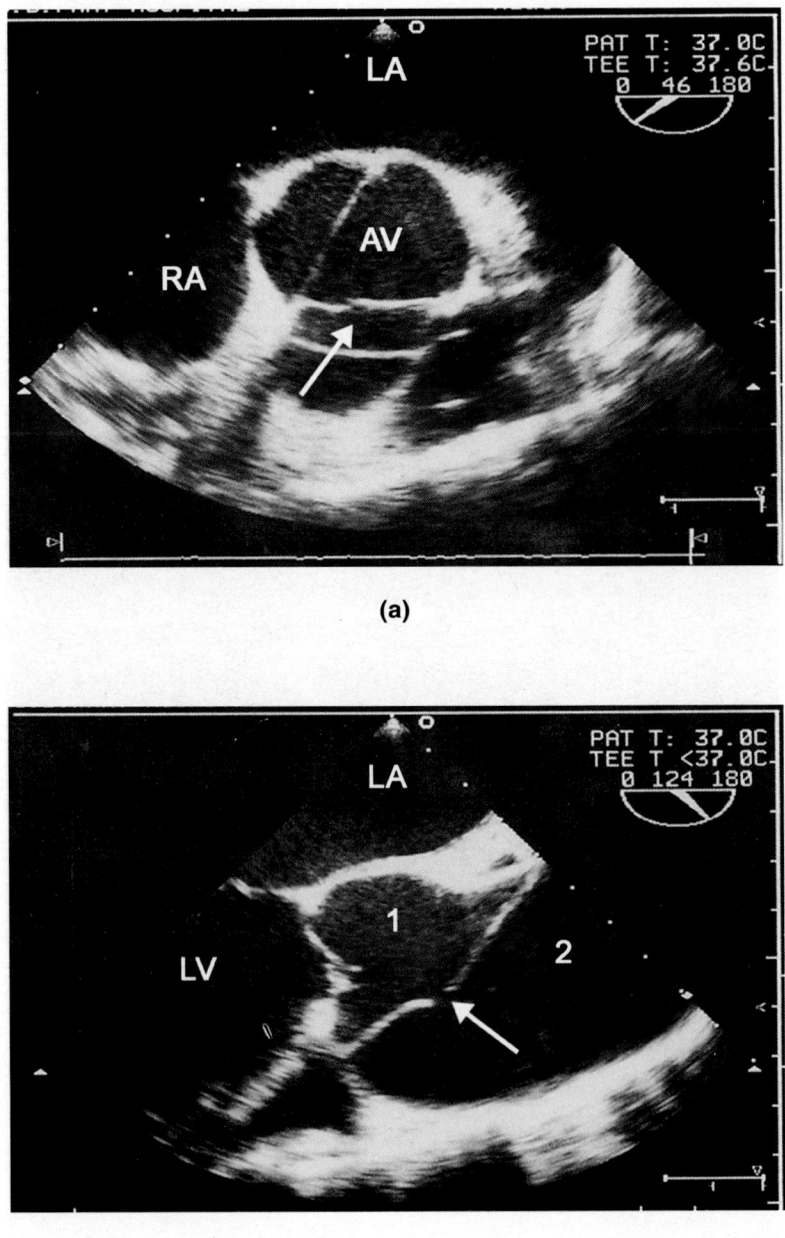

(a)

(b)

Figure 11.6. Trans-oesophageal echo in a patient with aortic dissection. Note the dissection flap (arrow) dividing the aortic lumen into true (1) and false lumens (2).(LA: left atrum, RA: right atrium, AV: aortic valve, LV: left ventricle)

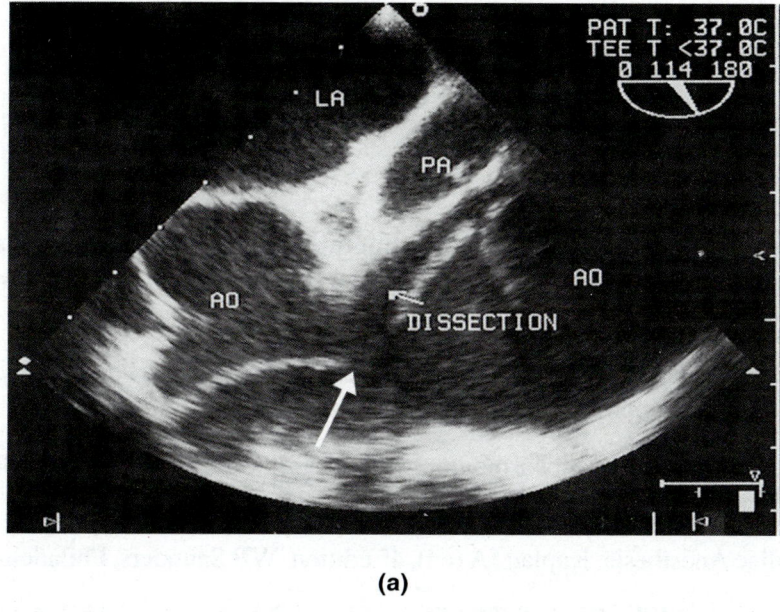

(a)

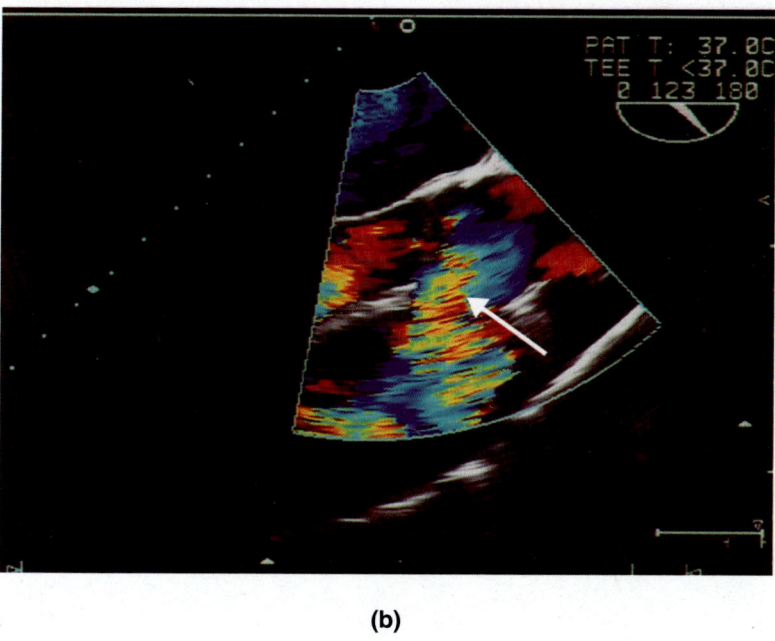

(b)

Figure 11.7 (a) The ascending aorta of a patient with aortic dissection. Note the entry point (arrow). **(b)** Colour flow shows blood flow in true and false lumen. (LA: left atrium, AO: aorta, PA: pulmonary artery)

Further Reading

1. Clinical Transesophageal echocardiography: A problem oriented approach, Konstadt SN, Sherman SK, Oka Y (editors), 2nd edition, Lippincott Williams & Wilkins, 2003.

2. A practical approach to Transesophageal echocardiography, Perrino AC Jr, Reeves ST (editors), Lippincott Williams & Wilkins, 2003.

3. Transoesophageal Echocardiography in Anaesthesia, Poelaert J and Skarvan K, (editors), BMJ Books, London, 2000.

4. Cardiac Anesthesia, Kaplan JA (ed), 4th edition, WB Saunders, Philadelphia, 1999.

5. Anesthesia, Miller RD (ed), 5th edition, Churchill Livingstone, Philadelphia, 2000.